Human Subjects Research

An Insider's View

Harry C. S. Wingfield, CIP

DEDICATION

For all the research participants, AIDS community activists, researchers, research team members, Institutional Review Board Members, and IRB team members I have had the pleasure of working with. A special dedication to my family: My husband, Vernon D. Push, who has listened to me rant about research since 1990 and to my siblings: Bitsy, Trip, Vera and Lou, who have always encouraged me to be my best.

CONTENTS

ACKNOWLEDGMENTS

Thank you to my husband Vern Push for encouraging me and putting up with me, to my sister Elizabeth Dick for valuable editing advice, to my sisters Lou Childs and Vera Stewart for being role models for successful business, and to my brother, Trip Wingfield, for being my biggest cheerleader.

INTRODUCTION

What is "Human Subjects Research?" The short answer is "research that involves people." Most of us know a little about Human Subjects Research. We might know that drugs must be approved by the FDA. We might have seen an ad on TV that says a drug is clinically proven to extend life or reduce symptoms. We have probably been asked to take a survey or complete a questionnaire. We may have signed a permission form that says we will let our medical records be used for research. But most of us don't know where research comes from, how it is conducted, who makes sure it is safe, or how the results are used.

When I was a kid, one of my mother's favorite expressions was "If you had seen the kitchen, you'd never want to eat there." She wasn't always talking about restaurants. She applied it to any entity that looked different when you went beyond what the average person sees and got a glimpse of what happens behind the scenes.

I have been a participant in medical research studies. My life was saved by one medical research study, and it was put in danger by mistakes made by doctors conducting two other medical research studies. I became an AIDS advocate, activist, and community representative. Then I went to work in an HIV research clinic, in charge of all the compliance paperwork.

From there I went to work for an Institutional Review Board, a committee that reviews and approves research involving humans. They look at the ethics of the study, and they also look for whether the study is consistent with Federal and local rules governing the conduct of research. They oversee the study throughout the life of the study, monitoring enrollment, changes in the research, any medical or other problems caused by the study, and any mistakes made by the study team. I became Board certified as a Certified IRB Professional.

I have seen research from many sides: as someone pressured to do research, as a research participant, as an advocate/activist for research participants, as a member of the research team that conducts research, and as a part of the oversight process. I can tell you what goes on behind the scenes.

I have seen research that has led to major improvements in medical care, including the study that saved my life. But I have also seen flaws in the way research is conducted, including some flaws that risked my health. These flaws include the motivation for doing the research, the lack of training for many research team members, and recruitment methods that bypassed the need to make sure the participants knew what they were signing up for.

By telling my story, I hope to help to identify areas where improvements are needed, and to offer my thoughts on how these improvements can be made. Along the way, I will teach you useful information about Human Subjects Research.

1 MY FIRST ENCOUNTERS WITH RESEARCH

- *Getting outed by research.*
- *Research required for an advanced degree in theatre.*
- *Tenure for university faculty requires published research*

Getting outed by research. My first experience with research involving humans came in the early 1970s. I was a student at the University of Georgia and joined a fraternity there. Our faculty advisor was working on his PhD in psychology. During my sophomore year, he came to one of the fraternity's monthly meetings to tell us about a research project he was working on. He needed our help as participants. The study goal was to see if the research team could find differences in the blood of gay men and straight men. He was hoping to find something in the genetic makeup to help predict who was gay and who was not gay. Almost everyone in the fraternity volunteered to take part.

On my appointment day, I met with the fraternity advisor, who was the main researcher on the study (principal investigator). I don't remember if I signed any kind of consent form. I must have, but I don't remember reading anything about potential risks, or about how my information would be kept confidential. He had me view some slides while he used a camera to record whether the iris in my eye got larger or smaller with each slide. Some of the slides were neutral: landscapes, art, crowd scenes. Some, however, were designed to see if there would be a sexual response. There were photos of nude women, and photos of nude men. There were close ups of genitals and other body parts like women's

3

breasts and men's muscles. There were photos of various types of sexual activities, involving various combinations of genders. I looked at the slides, and the machine measured the movement of my iris. Then the principal investigator drew some blood, gave me my gift card, and thanked me as I left his lab room.

A few weeks later he came back to the fraternity meeting. We thought he might have some results. Instead, he said he needed to re-test a few of us, and then, in front of the entire fraternity, he called out about six names of people he needed to re-test. There was a moment of silence, while we all simultaneously looked around the room and avoided eye contact. I was one of the names called. At that time, I didn't know for sure if I was gay. I certainly was not ready to have my fraternity brothers know this secret. I felt like the faculty advisor had violated my privacy. I had to put on a brave face and pretend it was not a big deal. All of us whose names were called were obviously upset, though.

Today, there are regulations in place to protect participants in studies like this. If a person decides to take part in a research study, they must be informed of all the potential risks, including physical risks like side effects, emotional risks, risks of loss of confidentiality, and others. Someone who wants to conduct research involving human participants must have the research plan approved by a committee called an Institutional Review Board or IRB. An IRB is an independent board made up of people from a variety of backgrounds. The IRB reviews studies to make sure risks are being minimized, and the rights of participants are being protected. An IRB must approve a research study before it begins. Reviews happen again before any changes are made to a study. In the case of the "gay gene" study, the investigator would now need to get the IRB to approve the plan to obtain additional information from some of the participants. A diligent IRB would recommend a better plan for informing the few participants from whom he needed additional information. This plan would need to ensure that the contact with these participants would be done using confidentiality, so that their personal information would remain private.

We were never told the results of the study. I imagine that if he had found any genetic markers for homosexuality, it would have been big news, and might have changed the way society viewed gay people. If being gay is not a choice, then maybe the moral objections to homosexuality would be diminished. I suspect the main reason we never found out about the results of the study is that the faculty advisor was doing the research project primarily to fulfill a requirement to get his PhD degree. If the primary goal of the study was to change the scientific view of why some people are gay, the study would have been done at multiple sites in a variety of geographic locations.

Later in this book I will talk about the types of research studies, including the differences between research done to increase scientific knowledge, and research done to fulfill degree requirements or to ensure job security. Currently, almost anyone pursuing an advanced degree, or wanting to work in an academic institution, must do research, even if they do not want to be a researcher. I found this out a few years later, when I was working on a master's degree in theatrical costume design at the University of Texas at Austin, and later when I was hired as a tenure-track assistant professor of theatre and dance at the University of Alabama at Birmingham.

<u>Research requirement for an advanced degree</u>. Who

knew that a costume designer needed to do research? I certainly did not. But when I reached the point in my Master of Fine Arts (MFA) degree program when I was ready to start on my final project, my advisor informed me I would need to write a research thesis as part of the project. Even though my thesis would not be considered human subjects research, I want to describe it here. It is an example of using a research requirement to teach a student how to be better at their chosen profession, rather than to become a researcher.

Anyone getting an advanced degree at the University of Texas had to write a research thesis. When the thesis was approved, a bound copy would be placed in the main library at the University of Texas. I had been assigned to design costumes for an upcoming production of a play by Edward Bond called Bingo. This was to be my final project for my MFA degree. I asked my advisor how my designs could be turned into a research project. He took me through my education history since I had started the MFA program three years earlier. I took courses in theatre history. The play, Bingo, was a fictional story about Shakespeare, so knowledge of theatre of Shakespeare's time was crucial to my design process and needed to be documented in my thesis. The play has a political viewpoint, exposing the mistreatment and criminalization of poverty-stricken people in Shakespeare's time. So I needed to research not only the author's political leanings, but also the political times in which the play was set, and the relevance of those times to the world of 1986, when the play was being presented at the University of Texas. During my degree program, I had taken courses in play analysis. As a designer, I needed to look at the themes of the play, the tone of the play, the type of language of the play, and the structure of the play. I had to study each character in the play, what they represented, who they were, and how they fit into the themes and structure of the play. All these things related to what the characters should look like. And all this had to be written down in my research thesis.

I researched previous productions of the play and looked at photographs from these productions. I met with the director to find out his interpretations of the play, and what artistic inspirations he wanted me to use. I consulted with the lighting, sound, and scenic designers to make sure all of us were working toward a harmonious goal.

Next, we moved into the actual construction of the costumes. At dress rehearsals, the scenic, lighting, sound designers and I worked together with the director to ensure we were presenting a unified vision. All this was documented in the research thesis.

During the run of the play, audience members were asked to fill out a short survey after each performance, which all the team members used to document the relative success of our contributions to the production.

While my research thesis was not primarily Human Subjects Research (research on people), the opinions and reviews I collected added a human subjects element to the research project. I spent a year from my initial project assignment until completion of the thesis. While the only tangible publication of my work was the bound copy of the thesis that went into the library, each performance of the play represented a form of "publication."

My work on this production of Edward Bond's Bingo would never be published in a professional journal, but my thesis documented my contribution to the creation of a work of art. One purpose of my research was to fulfill a degree requirement. However, the goal of that degree requirement was to make me a better costume designer, worthy to represent the theatre department of the University of Texas at Austin.

Research requirement for tenure. A few years later, I got my first tenure-track teaching job at the University of Alabama at Birmingham. The chairman of the theatre and dance department let me know that to get tenure, I would need to do research and have it published. I told him that I assumed that the costume design work that was part of my job description would meet the criteria for research and publication, since I always did the same kind of research I had done for my master's thesis for any theatrical design project. I also assumed that the production itself would be my publication. He told me that UAB (University of Alabama at Birmingham) took a much narrower view of research and publication, and that I would have to conduct scholarly research and have articles posted in professional journals. I was not aware of any professional journals on costume design. I did not make tenure in the UAB theatre and dance department. My contract was not renewed after my first two years, concurrently with my diagnosis with HIV and AIDS. This led to me becoming a research participant again.

2 RESEARCH PARTICIPANT

- *Sometimes research needs to be done that proves a problem exists before research can be done to find solutions to the problem.*
- *Even if the study drug or device turns out to not work well, important information for future research can be learned from the failure.*
- *Not everyone working in research has enough training to do their part in the research.*
- *There are outside factors, like financial incentives or the need for researchers to publish to advance their careers, that could impact how research is conducted.*
- *Informed consent forms are often not written with language that the average reader can easily understand and remember.*
- *Research that is not conducted properly can endanger the lives of the participants.*
- *Research that is not designed well can deprive participants of standard care and put their health at risk.*
- *IRBs sometimes approve studies that should not be approved.*
- *Patient payments can entice participants to take part in research that harms them.*
- *On the other hand, new drugs became available, because of research, that improved my health and probably saved my life.*
- *I still believe in research.*

Background and definitions. Before I talk about my experience as a participant in AIDS research, I want to provide a brief overview of the types of research that can be done.

Many types of activities fall under the umbrella of "research." At the lowest risk level is "Not Human Subjects Research" or "NHSR." Like my master's thesis, and the scholarly work I might have done on clothing history, these projects do not involve human subjects according to the definitions provided by the NIH (National Institutes of Health) and the OHRP (Office of Human Research Protections). Together, these two agencies define research as "A systematic investigation, including research development, testing and evaluation, designed to develop or contribute to generalizable knowledge." Human subjects are defined by the department of Health and Human Services as:

"a living individual about whom an investigator (whether professional or student) conducting research:

- Obtains information or biospecimens through intervention or interaction with the individual, and uses, studies, or analyzes the information or biospecimens; or
- Obtains, uses, studies, analyzes, or generates identifiable private information or identifiable biospecimens."

Research that does not meet the definition of "research" AND the definition of "human subjects" is Not Human Subjects Research. This category of research does not need to be approved by the Institutional Review Board (IRB), an entity designed to protect research participants. However, other departments at an institution may need to give the OK to do this kind of research project.

Research that meets criteria for very minimal risk to participants can be classified as "Exempt Review." This means it is not subject to IRB review. However, most institutions rely on someone from the IRB or the IRB staff to make the final decision on whether the research qualifies as Exempt Review.

Research that carries some risks, most commonly the risk of loss of confidentiality and other risks that are considered "minimal," falls under the category of <u>Expedited Review</u>. This means that the IRB must approve the research, but that this approval process can be done by a single person rather than requiring review and approval by the entire Board.

Any human subjects research that is more than minimal risk must be approved at a formal meeting of the Institutional Review Board. This is called <u>Full Board Review</u>.

Detailed descriptions of these research review levels can be found in the Code of Federal Regulations. A Google search for "Human Subjects Research categories" will take you to lists that are easily read and understood. These lists found in the Google search are from web sites for IRBs at universities and hospitals that conduct research.

When a new drug is developed, the research is usually done in phases.

- Phase I research is done to establish whether the drug is safe, and to determine the highest possible dose of the drug that can be given without causing too many side effects. The first few patients will get a dose that would likely not be strong enough to have any benefit. The next few patients get a stronger dose. This continues until the dose given causes unacceptable side effects. When that happens, the researchers usually go back to the previous dose and use it for further research. Phase I research usually only looks at drug safety and does not look at whether the drug is effective in treating the condition. Because of this, Phase I studies usually enroll healthy volunteers, like college students who need some extra money. Sometimes, though, the researchers need to establish drug safety and the highest acceptable dose in patients who have the disease. For conditions like cancer or HIV, Phase I research may enroll patients who have the disease, have not responded to any approved treatments, and have no other treatment options. Even though these participants are not likely to benefit from the Phase I study, many will enroll out of a desire to help provide better treatments for future patients.

- Phase II research proceeds once Phase I research proves the drug is safe enough to use. Phase II research will use the "optimal dose" (highest acceptable dose) that was established in Phase I. In Phase II, the researchers begin to look at whether the drug will work in treating the illness. The enrollments are still small, but are larger than the enrollments in Phase I. Phase II no longer needs healthy volunteers to enroll, since the safety of the drug has been established. Phase II collects data on whether the drug can benefit patients who have the condition being treated.

- Phase III begins if the results from Phase II are favorable. Phase III studies will enroll large numbers of participants at many locations. Phase III studies usually compare the experimental drug with either a placebo (a substance that looks like the experimental drug but has no active ingredients) or an approved treatment, or with both a placebo and an approved treatment. Patients are randomized (assigned by chance) to one of the treatments that are being compared. At the end of Phase III, researchers should have data to prove that the new drug works better than placebo, and either works as well as or works better than the approved drug or drugs. If the results from Phase III are favorable, the researchers will submit the study results to the FDA, so that the FDA can decide whether to approve the drug. Sometimes the FDA approves the drug but requires additional research to support the approval. If the Phase III results are favorable enough, and the disease to be treated is serious enough, the FDA can issue an accelerated approval. Accelerated approval means the drug can be prescribed because it is likely to benefit patients, even if more data is needed.

- Phase IV studies are done when the FDA wants more data to confirm an accelerated approval. For most Phase IV studies, patients who are prescribed the newly approved drug are asked to participate, so their data can be collected and sent to the FDA. Occasionally the FDA will require that any patient who is prescribed the newly approved drug must enroll in the Phase IV study in order to receive the drug.

Participant in AIDS research. As soon as I was diagnosed with AIDS, I was asked to take part in research studies. Some of these were minimal risk/expedited review, like survey studies, or focus groups that discussed various topics. Since the HIV clinic at UAB is a major clinical research clinic, I was also asked to enroll in research studies that were more than minimal risk. Some of these were testing new treatments for HIV. Some were looking for better ways to handle side effects of HIV medications. Others were testing drugs that would treat or prevent the kinds of serious infections that were likely to occur in people living with HIV and AIDS.

As my medical records at the UAB AIDS clinic grew, it is likely that my data was used in research (called "chart review" research) that I was never made aware of. I had signed a general consent form when I became a patient at the clinic. The form stated that I agreed to allow my medical records at the clinic to be used for research purposes. I did not know it at the time, but all these chart review projects had to be reviewed and approved by the UAB IRB. The person at the IRB who approved these projects checked to make sure my personal data would be protected, and that only the minimal amount of data needed to do the research would be used.

I also enrolled in more than minimal risk studies. For these,

I signed an informed consent form and was made aware that I was going to be taking part in a research study. The consent form for each study informed me:

- The study involved research
- The reason I was being invited to take part,
- The purpose of the research study
- What would happen in the study
- Which parts of the study were experimental
- The risks of taking part
- If there might be any benefits to me or others if I took part
- How my confidentiality would be protected
- Who would have access to my private information
- Whether there would be any compensation if I got injured because of taking part in the study
- Who to contact if I had questions or concerns
- What my alternatives would be if I did not want to take part
- That I could withdraw from the study at any time, with no penalty to me
- Under what circumstances I might be removed from the study
- Taking part in the study was entirely voluntary
- If taking part in the study might involve additional costs to me
- I would be informed if any new information became available that might affect my willingness to take part
- What I would need to do when the study ended, or when I decided not to continue.
- Whether or not I would find out about the results of the study when it was completed.

I was also told that I would receive a copy of the signed consent form for my records and for future reference.

The informed consent forms I signed for research in the early

1990s were not easy to understand. They contained words and phrases that seemed to come from medical experts and/or lawyers. A lot of my friends said they trusted their doctor, and just glanced over the form before signing it.

I trusted my doctor, too, but I did not necessarily trust whoever designed the study. Some of the studies were developed and funded by the government through the National Institutes of Health. Others were developed and funded by for-profit drug companies or medical device companies. A few were designed by a doctor at my hospital and may or may not have had any outside funding. So even though I trusted my doctor, I still wanted to be sure what I was signing up for before I put my name on the form.

I asked questions.

"This says I can withdraw from the study at any time without penalty. Is that right? Why would I want to withdraw? Is the clinic really not going to hold a grudge if I don't fulfill my commitment?"

"I don't know what some of these risks are."

"What is nephrolithiasis?" It was kidney stones.

"What is dyspnea?" It was trouble breathing.

"What is thrombocytopenia?" It was low platelets in the blood, which could cause excessive bleeding.

The list went on and on. I was a little angry that this document, which was supposed to be telling me enough about the study so I could make my own decision about whether to enroll, was so hard to understand. I'm a fairly intelligent person and have scored high on reading comprehension tests. I wondered what would happen to others who might not have my ability to understand and retain this kind of information.

When I was first diagnosed with AIDS, the only approved treatment was a drug called AZT. Several of my friends had been in the research studies that were done to get FDA approval for AZT. In some of these studies, participants got doses of the drug that caused serious side effects. The companies that develop the drugs have to expose some patients to these risks, so that they can determine how much of the drug they can give a patient without exposing the patient to too much toxicity. Several of my friends had gotten permanent liver damage from taking part in the early AZT studies. Other friends who took part in these studies got a dose that was not high enough to control the HIV in their bodies. For these friends, their virus quickly became resistant to the HIV, and the drug no longer worked for them. This made me very careful about what studies I signed up for.

The "L-drug." The first study I enrolled in, several months after I was diagnosed, was for an early version of a new drug that would fight HIV in a different way than AZT did. I had already developed resistance to AZT and no longer took it, because I would still get the serious side effects without any benefit from the drug. The AIDS community was finding out that even with the best dose of AZT, eventually the virus would mutate, and the drug would no longer work.

Those of us that signed up for this new study, looking at a drug we called the "L-drug," were informed that any benefit from this drug might not be permanent, but that the medical community could learn information from the studies that might help develop better drugs in the future. Even with that risk, I decided to enroll in the study. So many of my friends were dying from HIV. I figured if the study could buy me a little more time, that would be good enough.

As it turned out, the L-drug worked great, for a few weeks or less, and then the effects vanished. If I remember right, this study was done when researchers had just learned how to measure the amount of virus in the body, or "viral load."

Almost everyone in the study saw their viral load go down dramatically, and then go back up. For some of us it went to higher levels than it was before we started the study.

Was the study a failure? Not completely. The researchers found out that the benefits of the drug, when taken by itself, did not last. But they also used data collected in the study to find out for the first time how rapidly the individual virus cells multiplied.

Each virion, or virus cell, could multiply about a million times in one day. This is why a single drug could not work well for very long. If anything multiplies that many times in one day, the chances of a mutation are high. Some of those mutations might weaken the virus, others might make it more dangerous. The important mutation for AIDS research was the mutation which made the virus immune to the current treatment. Even if only one such mutant virion was immune, it could multiply a million times, very quickly, while all the other virus cells were being suppressed by the treatment. Soon the person's body would be overtaken by the "offspring" of the mutant virus, and the drug would no longer work.

That was the major finding from the L-drug study. Researchers would have to develop a way of treating HIV with more than one drug at a time, with drugs that suppressed virus replication in different parts of the virus life cycle, in order for the virus to remain suppressed over time.

CMV suppression (prophylaxis) study. Some of the studies I enrolled in were for preventing the "opportunistic infections" that became likely in patients whose immune system was repressed. One such infection that was feared in the HIV/AIDS community was CMV (Cytomegalovirus), which could attack the retina in the eyes and make you go blind. To enroll in the study, you had to have evidence of CMV in your blood stream, but no active CMV infections. I knew I had recently been exposed to CMV. The tests I took to see if I was eligible for the study confirmed that I had CMV in my blood stream, so I agreed to take part.

Participants would take the drug or a placebo daily for many months, possibly years. The research would look for how long it took for each participant to develop CMV related symptoms, and then compare the results from those who took the experimental drug with those who took placebo. Once a month, I had to go to an ophthalmologist who would dilate my eyes and look for any signs of CMV retinitis. I took my pill three times a day – first thing in the morning, at around 2:00 in the afternoon, and just before bedtime. I did not know if I was getting the drug or the placebo. I did notice some side effects like nausea, diarrhea, and headaches, so I thought I was probably getting the real test drug.

One afternoon, about fifteen minutes before it was time for me to take my pill, the phone rang. It was my study nurse. He asked if I had taken my afternoon pill yet. I told him I had not. He yelled "DON'T TAKE IT!!!" I put the pill bottle down and asked him what was going on.

He explained that while he didn't know if I was getting drug or placebo, and the doctor didn't know if I was getting the drug or placebo, there was a group of scientists and physicians who were not part of the study team who did have access to that information. They looked at the results of the study at pre-determined time points to see if risks to all participants were being minimized. If they could see, while the study was in progress, that there were significantly higher health benefits in the group that was getting the test drug, when compared to the group that was getting placebo, this would mean that there was increased risk to the placebo group.

The monitoring group, called a Data Safety Monitoring Committee or DSMB, might recommend that the data be unblinded. Unblinded means the researchers and the participants would find out who was getting the test drug and who was getting the placebo. The DSMB might also recommend that the study continue, with all participants given the option of getting the test drug.

In the CMV prevention study, however, the interim results when the DSMB looked at the data were not good. My study nurse told me that the interim analysis (the data at the predetermined timepoint) showed that more people died who were getting the test drug when compared to those getting placebo. The difference in the death rate was significant enough that the study was cancelled immediately. The researchers never found out if the drug would help prevent CMV disease, but it did find out that the side effects of the drug were too dangerous for the drug to continue in development. All the participants in the study were asked to come back to the clinic, bring all the pills we still had on hand, and have a thorough health check to see how the study had affected our health.

While I had been put at risk by taking part in the study, it was a risk that had been described well in the consent process, including the informed consent form that I had read and signed. I knew in advance that results like this might happen. The study team and the DSMB had worked well to make sure the risks to me were kept to a minimum.

Nutrition supplement study. Another study I took part in was for treatment of a common AIDS complication called "wasting syndrome." A lot of people who were living with AIDS were losing too much weight too fast. For the first few years after my diagnosis, this was not an issue for me. But as I started getting sicker, my weight went from over 180 pounds down to about 140 pounds. No matter how much I ate, or how many calories I consumed, I couldn't keep the weight on. Some research had already been done on the causes of this wasting syndrome. One theory was that our digestive systems were no longer able to absorb fat. If we ate a fatty diet, it moved through our system quickly, causing severe diarrhea. Our bodies did not give our digestive systems enough time to absorb any nutrients from the food we were eating.

Some nutritionists had a theory that if a nutrition supplement could be developed with a kind of fat called "medium chain triglycerides" (MCT) instead of "long chain triglycerides" this would help with our ability to absorb nutrition from our foods. Since I had wasting syndrome, I was asked to take part in a study comparing a standard nutrition supplement with one based on MCT. I had to check into the hospital's research unit, which at the time was called the GCRC, or General Clinical Research Center.

I was put into a hospital room. I was told I could not leave that room for the two weeks of the study. The study team measured everything that went into my body, and everything that came out. My water glass was monitored to measure how much water I drank. I urinated into a container which was measured and weighed every day. I pooped into a container which was also measured and weighed every day. I was only allowed to consume three "meals" a day, with nothing in between.

Each meal consisted of a tall glass of a milkshake-like drink. It was either a commercially available nutrition supplement, something like Boost or Ensure, or it was the study drink. I had the choice of vanilla, chocolate, or strawberry. I chose chocolate.

The study paid each participant about $2,000 for our time on the study. Since I was on disability income at the time, this was a powerful incentive to take part. I went over the informed consent form with the study coordinator and the study doctor before I was enrolled in the study. I asked a lot of questions, and got the doctor to agree to let me take walks inside the hospital every day so I could keep getting some exercise, as long as I never left the building and promised not to eat or drink or go to the bathroom while I was out walking.

I also got permission to bring my computer to the hospital so I could work on a play I was writing while I was confined to my room. I signed the informed consent form and took my copy home so I could study it some more before I went into the hospital for the study.

During the consent process, before I signed, I asked the study doctor about my recent illness with an infection called c-diff or c-difficile. The long name for the disease is Clostridium Difficile. It is extremely contagious and hard to treat. It produces severe, painful inflammation of the colon, resulting in severe diarrhea and bloody stools. It can be fatal if not successfully treated. My study doctor said that enough time had passed since I last had any symptoms, and I should be OK to enroll in the study. Looking back at my experience with additional knowledge I have picked up in my work in research and research oversight, I wonder now if my previous c-diff infection should have been an exclusion which would have prevented me from taking part in the study. I have no way of knowing that now. If it was an exclusion, the study team overlooked it.

After a few days of drinking milkshakes and pooping in a bucket, I started having severe cramping in my abdomen. I developed diarrhea and noticed there was some blood in my stools. I wondered if this was a side effect of the milkshakes. I pulled out my copy of the consent form from by computer bag, and double checked the risk list to see if the extreme diarrhea or the bloody stools were a known risk. They were not listed in the consent form. I was worried that my c-diff infection might be coming back.

Remembering how sick I had been before, and how worried my doctors were, I asked the study doctor to send a sample of my stool to the lab to be tested. He said he couldn't do that, because the study team had to save all the specimens for the sponsor, in case they were needed in the future for further research.

I told the doctor that if I couldn't get my stool tested for c-diff, that I would have to leave the study so I could see my primary doctor. The study doctor said "You can't leave the study! You signed a consent form." I once again pulled out my copy of the signed consent form, and showed him the paragraph that said "You have the right to withdraw from this research study at any time, with no penalty to you." His face turned white, and he agreed to send a small sample of my stool for testing, and mark in my study chart that a portion of that day's stool was missing from the stored sample due to the need for c-diff testing.

I wondered if he had been trained on the study. I wondered if he had been trained in conducting research, since the right of the participant to withdraw from a study at any time is part of every research study. I wondered if he was aware that I had this right but was hoping I didn't know. I wondered if the doctor didn't want me to leave the study because he was getting money for the number of patients who completed the study. I also wondered what might have happened to me if I was not the kind of person who read everything I signed, asked a lot of questions, and kept a copy of signed documents in my files so that I could look at them later if I needed to.

The tests for c-diff came back negative. I should have left the study anyway. If I did not have c-diff, that meant the diet that I was on was the cause of my severe bloody diarrhea. But I wanted that money. I completed the study and received my $2,000. I never found out the results of the study. The large payment for participation was a major incentive for me to take part in the study.

Even though I qualified for the study due to my diagnosis of wasting syndrome, I had been able to maintain good nutrition before entering the study by carefully watching my diet and avoiding foods with high fat content. I gave up my ability to control my diet when I agreed to take part in the study. No one on the study received a balanced diet of low fat solid foods, only the milkshakes.

Looking back on this experience, I now believe the IRB should not have approved the study. Participants were being denied standard care because we were denied an optimal diet. It is likely that neither the commercially available nutrition supplement nor the test product provided adequate nutrition.

Even approved nutritional supplements are not intended to completely replace other foods. I lost more weight while I was on the study. My health declined. I lost muscle strength. It took me years to get my health back to where it had been before I took part in the study. My wasting syndrome eventually went away, once I got on better treatments for my AIDS and made some changes to my diet. Then I was able to start exercising again and getting my strength back.

The nutrition study was not the only research being done at the GCRC. Down the hall from my room was a room with newborns who picked up CMV infections from their mothers during the birth process. I believe the study they were on was testing which CMV treatments would be safest in newborns. Because the newborns were so delicate, treatment of this dangerous virus was essential. The nurse who came in three times a day to check my vital signs was also working with the sick babies down the hall. I would often see her walking with one of the babies, gently speaking to the baby and rocking it in her arms to calm it down. Then she would come directly to my room to check my blood pressure and temperature. I asked her if she had washed her hands after she handled the baby. She was not wearing a mask or gloves. She got very offended when I asked the question and did not answer. It was a few weeks later that I found out I had CMV in my blood and was asked to take part in the CMV prophylaxis study I described earlier.

I wondered how much training in disease prevention the

GCRC nurse had completed. I wondered if she had gotten any training on my study, so that she could know that I had almost no immune system and had to be protected from exposure to other diseases. I wondered if my study team was aware of the dangers to the participants in the AIDS nutrition study because of the poor clinical practices of the GCRC nurse.

HPV vaccine study. I was in another study a few years later, after I had gone back to work in the research clinic. This study was developed by my primary doctor in the AIDS clinic and his nurse practitioner. At the time, companies like Merck were in the final stages of developing vaccines for young girls to take, that would prevent them from contracting HPV (Human Papillomavirus) when they got older. HPV is known to contribute to the risks of developing some kinds of cancer, so the vaccine could help prevent these cancers. My doctor and nurse felt that some men, especially gay men, could also benefit from the vaccine.

Before widespread research can be done to develop a treatment for a problem, researchers first must prove that the problem exists. That was the goal of this study, to find out if gay men were also exposed to HPV which could cause cancer. They were asking their male HIV patients to take part in a study that would look for the presence of HPV and see if this HPV might be linked to cancers in men, the way it is linked to cancer in women. Since I had some experience in writing and editing consent forms for federally funded AIDS research, they asked me to edit their consent form to make sure it was readable and gave an accurate description of the proposed study.

The main part of the study required each patient to have a procedure called a sigmoidoscopy. A sigmoidoscopy is similar to a colonoscopy, but the scope they use to examine your intestines doesn't go as far in, so general anesthesia is not required. A sigmoidoscopy is used to check for ulcers, abnormal cells, and polyps. The GI (gastrointestinal) doctor who would conduct the sigmoidoscopy would also take a swab of the colon. The swab would be used to check for the presence of HPV, similar to the way a "pap smear" in women is used to check for diseases.

As I reviewed the consent form, I noticed that the GI doctor would only take a biopsy specimen if he saw abnormal tissue while looking at the inside of the colon during the sigmoidoscopy. I checked the protocol to make sure the consent form language was consistent with the procedures in the protocol. Then I asked my doctor and nurse if this was what they intended. They confirmed that not every participant would get a biopsy, only the ones with abnormal tissue. This was important to me because a close friend, a woman with AIDS, was clinging to life because of complications from a perforated intestine. I knew that any procedure that would take a bit of tissue from the wall of the intestine could be serious and should not be done unless there was disease present that needed to be diagnosed.

I enrolled in the study. I made several appointments with the GI doctor for my sigmoidoscopy, but they were cancelled. This was frustrating because I had to request a day off from work at my clinic to have the procedure. I found out that since the GI doctor was not getting paid as much for the study participants as he was for his regular patients, he was cancelling the study appointments if he had a regular patient to see instead.

After three or four cancelled appointments, I finally got my sigmoidoscopy. I was awake during the entire procedure and could see what the camera in the scope saw as it went inside me. I was lying on the procedure table, barely covered with a hospital gown that did not cover my rear end. The doctor walked in followed by ten or twelve others wearing scrubs and masks. He explained that they were medical students who were there to observe the procedure. I had not consented to this. I should have been asked beforehand if I was OK with having an audience. When the doctor told me who the observers were, he may or may not have asked me if I minded being observed. Even if he had asked, I was not in a position (literally or figuratively) to object at that time. I had finally gotten an appointment and wanted to get it over with. The students could look at my butt all they wanted to.

The GI doctor started the procedure, making sure the students and I could see the monitor. He took a swab of the lining of my colon and passed this on to an assistant to prepare for testing. The scope went further in, with the doctor making "um humm" noises along the way. Then he spoke to the students: "This patient's colon looks fine, but since he is a research participant, I'm going to take a biopsy now." I asked him if he saw any abnormal tissue. He said no, but he was taking a biopsy from all the research participants. I thought to myself "You don't know who you are talking to!" I told him I had helped write the consent form for the study and knew that he was not supposed to take a biopsy from participants with no visible sign of disease. He did not respond. I watched the screen as the end of the scope opened and cut a chunk of tissue out of my large intestine. I watched the stream of blood float away from the biopsy site. The scope was pulled out of me, the doctor covered my butt with the hospital gown, and walked out of the procedure room, followed by the medical students.

As soon as I could, I went to the AIDS clinic and found my nurse practitioner who helped write the study. I told him what had happened. He called my AIDS doctor, the primary investigator on the study, and told him. They both apologized and assured me it would not happen again. The error was made because the GI doctor, who was part of the study team, either did not get sufficient education on the study procedures or got the education and either forgot or ignored it. I should have called the IRB and reported the protocol deviation. But I did not want the study to get shut down. I wanted the results to be completed and published. I wanted for young boys to get the same benefit from the HPV vaccine as young girls were getting. The study found that gay men are at risk for HPV infections and that this infection can lead to pre-cancerous conditions and then to cancer in some patients. The vaccine is now marketed to all children, not just young girls. But a lot of men with HIV and AIDS in Birmingham had gotten an unnecessary invasive procedure along the way, because the GI doctor did not follow the protocol.

Expanded access program. The UAB AIDS Research clinic also saved my life, by opening an expanded access program for a new drug called Indinavir. Expanded access programs are not designed as research studies, although the study may collect some information on the participants. They are designed mainly to provide access to a drug that has shown benefit in clinical trials, and is close to FDA approval, but is not yet FDA approved. Because the drug is still considered "investigational," the expanded access programs are usually done in research clinics. They require approval by an Institutional Review Board before patients can start taking the drug.

Normally the only way to have access to a drug that is not approved by the FDA is to enroll in a research study or clinical trial. But not everyone lives near enough to a research center to be able to enroll in a study. Not everyone meets the eligibility criteria to enroll in a study. When a drug company is trying to get FDA approval for a drug, they want to enroll patients who have the disease being treated, but don't have a whole lot of other health problems. This keeps the data clean and helps show if the results of the study are related only to the new drug being tested. If they enrolled people who had multiple health problems in addition to AIDS, then if the participant died from one of the other health problems, the study results would still show a high death rate from people who got the drug, even if the death was not related to the drug.

I was one of those people who was too sick to enroll in the clinical trial for Indinavir. I had wasting syndrome. I had almost no immune system. I had tested positive for CMV. I had been hospitalized four times for Pneumocystis pneumonia (PCP), also known as "AIDS pneumonia." I could barely walk more than half a block.

UAB was one of the highest enrolling sites for the Indinavir research studies. Because of their good relationship with Merck, the drug company that was developing Indinivir, the UAB AIDS Research clinic was chosen to be one of the first sites to open an expanded access program. My doctor called me to come to the clinic. I was one of the first to enroll. Because of my experience in the L-drug study, I had avoided trying all the other newer AIDS drugs on the market. They were all in the same class of drugs as AZT and worked the same way. Because they were usually prescribed as a single drug, I was afraid my virus would develop resistance, the way it had become resistant to AZT and to the L-drug. I wanted to wait until there was a new class of drugs that I could take along with one or two other AIDS medicines, to improve my chances of not developing drug resistance. The Indinivir expanded access program provided that opportunity.

I was put on Indinivir and two other drugs, a nucleoside reverse transcriptase inhibitor (similar to AZT) and a non-nucleoside reverse transcriptase inhibitor (a newer type of AIDS treatment). The tests to see if my virus was already resistant to these drugs were not yet available. My medical team and I crossed our fingers that it would work. I started the new drug "cocktail" the next day.

Within a week, I felt much better. I had more energy. I could walk a block or walk up a flight of stairs and not lose my breath. My appetite returned. I gained a few pounds. My medical team said I looked like Lazarus coming back from the dead. My virus never developed resistance to these new drugs. Within a few weeks, my viral load (the amount of virus in my body) went from astronomical figures to under 400 copies per mL. This was the lowest number the current tests could detect. The viral load might have been lower, but the tests available then could not test below 400. My immune system did not respond right away, but without having to fight the AIDS by itself, my body was better able to fight against the other health problems I was having. Many of my friends had died before the combination therapy became available. My improving health status allowed me to get more involved in AIDS research, as a community advocate for people living with AIDS, and as an activist.

Other research. I have participated in several other research studies. When people with AIDS started complaining that the new treatments were causing body shape changes, there was a major study comparing people on AIDS treatments with demographically matched HIV negative volunteers to see if the body changes were more extreme in people living with AIDS. I took part in this study. I was in a study to see if AIDS or AIDS treatment was associated with reduced mental capacity. I took part in an interview and survey study on the effects of aging in people with HIV and AIDS. When my medical treatment required a lymph node biopsy, I signed an informed consent form that allowed some of the lymph node tissue to be used for research purposes.

Over the years, I have taken part in many research studies that did not require a medical intervention. I have participated in survey studies on topics like my sexual history and my issues with aging and being HIV positive. I have participated in focus groups on recommendations for reaching a wider range of demographics when recruiting study participants. I have participated in studies of alternative medicine, from spiritual healing methods like Reiki and therapeutic touch, music therapy, art therapy and journaling.

3 COMMUNITY ADVOCATE AND ACTIVIST

- *From my participation in the Adult AIDS Clinical Trials group, I learned the importance of setting priorities for research, so that limited resources could be used in the most effective way. Not every research proposal got funded and developed.*
- *Providing federal funds for research allows research to get done that would not be possible if funding were dependent on industry that is mostly interested in profits.*
- *Representation of the community that will participate in the studies ensures the community's needs are being met. These needs include research that impacts current health issues and informed consent forms that clearly explain the purpose, procedures, and risks of the research.*

Background. In the early days of the AIDS epidemic, groups like ACT-UP (AIDS Coalition to Unleash Power) and its offshoot groups worked in powerful and creative ways to demand better treatment for HIV and AIDS, and to speed up and improve the process for developing these drugs. People with AIDS did not have the luxury of time. We needed better drugs NOW, because we were in danger of dying quickly once we were sick enough to be diagnosed. One of the changes the community activists demanded was that people representing the AIDS community be given a chair at the table. We wanted community input at all levels of AIDS research, from the allocation of funds to research, to the development of research studies, to the oversight of the research, to the local participation and conduct in research, to the publication of the results.

Community Advisory Boards. I got my AIDS diagnosis and went on disability at about the time the demands of ACT

UP and others were being addressed. The immediate impact on me came at the local level. The AIDS Research clinic at UAB had been invited to join a network for federally funded AIDS research clinics called the Adult AIDS Clinical Trials Group, or AACTG. One of the requirements of the AACTG was that each clinic must have a Community Advisory Board or CAB. The local CAB participated in the selection of research to be done at the clinic. We gave input on whether we thought the research was needed in our local community and if the design of the research was fair to the participants. At the UAB AIDS Research clinic, we were not just a figurehead group to satisfy network funding requirements. Our opinions were actively sought and respected by the researchers in the clinics. I accepted the request to be the chair of our local CAB. As the chair, I got an expense paid trip to the national conferences of the AACTG and got to see how the national CAB participated in setting research agendas, selecting which ideas would become research studies, deciding how these studies would be designed, and making sure the informed consent forms accurately represented the study procedures and risks, in a format that would be readable and understandable.

After serving at the local CAB chair for two years, I was invited to join the national AACTG CAB. This invitation did not come easy. The national CAB was dominated by people from New York City, San Francisco, and other major urban areas. Some of these people were not living with HIV or AIDS but were representing the AIDS community for the AACTG. The national CAB seemed reluctant to diversify the membership to include representation from all over the country. Since I was living in Birmingham, Alabama, I couldn't help but believe that some preconceived notions about the ignorance of southerners was preventing me from being selected. The group was also under pressure to include more women and more people of color. As a gay white male, my demographics were too similar to the demographics of others who were already on the Board. But I persevered, made my case well, and was eventually selected. Once I was selected, I was able to quickly demonstrate my value to the CAB.

<u>Setting priorities.</u> At the time I joined, the AACTG had three main areas of research. Each had its own Research Agenda Committee, or RAC. The three RACs were for drug treatment studies, studies on complications of AIDS and AIDS treatments, and studies on immune based treatments. Each RAC, on an annual basis, set priorities for the types of research it planned to fund that year, and published requests for proposals for new research ideas that fit these pre-established priorities.

As the RACs developed their annual priorities, the community members in the CAB meetings set priorities for what research was important to the people living with HIV and AIDS. These were not always the same as what the researchers on the RACs wanted to fund and study, but the powerful lobbying of the community members helped the community research goals get included.

For the RAC setting drug research priorities, the community members lobbied for studies on drugs that would have less serious side effects, and for new classes of drugs for patients whose virus was resistant to the available drugs.

For the RAC working on complications of AIDS and AIDS treatment, the community was interested in studies on the body shape changes many of us were seeing in ourselves and our friends. We were also interested in more research on the best way to treat patients who were co-infected with HIV and Hepatitis B (HBV) and/or Hepatitis C (HCV).

For the RAC working on immune based treatments, we were especially interested in a novel idea for having patients take periodic "drug holidays" in which they would go off their AIDS treatments for a specified period of time, sometimes with an immune boosting drug like IL-2. The researchers theorized that if the drugs were temporarily halted, the patient's own immune system would kick in again to help fight the HIV. So far, these studies had not worked. Some even sped up the process of viral resistance to the drugs they were taking. The researchers, though, were convinced that they needed to keep trying different drug holiday intervals and different immune boosting drugs until they found the one that would work. The community felt that they were putting science over patient safety. The community representation on that RAC kept patient safety as a priority when studies were selected for funding and development. Eventually, the AACTG reduced their interest in funding this type of research. Treatment interruption research was no longer a priority. The community input made a significant impact on this decision.

The AACTG CAB selected one voting member for each RAC. I was selected to be the community representative for the Complications RAC. I was also the community representative for the sub-RAC that looked at studies for patients co-infected with HIV, HBV and/or HCV. Within each RAC, once study proposals were selected for funding and development, each selected protocol team had to include one voting team member from the CAB. I served on at least ten protocol committees.

I was impressed with the research selection process. Each year, many more study proposals were submitted than we had funding for. Studies that fit the research priorities got more consideration. Studies that duplicated research already being done, or competed with existing studies for patients, were removed from consideration. As the community representative, I kept the community's interests at the forefront, and also provided advice, based on my experience as a research participant and as the local CAB chair, on what aspects of the research design might cause problems. Were they asking for too many clinic visits? Were painful invasive tests like colonoscopies or spinal taps being done when the same information could be obtained with a less risky or less invasive test? Were any groups being unnecessarily excluded from the study?

Many of the member sites in the AACTG were also conducting research overseas in underdeveloped countries, using AACTG funds. One requirement that was set for these studies is that the research must be done on drugs that would be available and affordable for the local population once the research was completed. A study being done in Zambia, for instance, could not use drugs that were not on the formulary for the Zambia health agencies. The unavailability of a drug could be either due to the drug not being approved for marketing in that country, or due to the drug being too expensive for the local health agencies to afford to provide it.

Some U.S. activists criticized the studies, because they were only studying drugs that had been deemed inferior in the developed world because of being less effective or having too many serious side effects. Others argued that testing newer drugs was putting research risks on a group that would not see any benefit from the results of the study. The newer drug might be better but would not be available for patients in that country once the study was over. Some of us wondered if the same standards should be applied to AACTG research in the United States. If the drugs we were helping to develop were going to be so expensive that insurance companies might not cover them, or cover them only with a copayment higher than most AIDS patients could afford, were we placing research patients at risk in the research when they would not be able to reap the benefits of the approved drug?

The committee also evaluated whether there was enough background information on a problem to justify conducting a treatment study. One community priority that was continually held back by this was the issue of breast enlargement in HIV positive women. For some women, the condition caused embarrassment or discomfort. We wanted to see if the breast enlargement was associated with specific HIV treatments or treatment combinations. The researchers countered that they could not fund this research without first getting scientific evidence that the problem of breast enlargement existed and was prevalent. The only evidence they had seen was anecdotal. One or two patients might complain about noticeable breast enlargement. But there were no "before" measurements to compare to current measurements. There were no data on other factors, like weight gain, that might cause the appearance of breast enlargement even if there was no additional enlargement happening. One researcher on the committee said: "We can't do the research to establish the problem because we don't have a scientifically valid way to measure breasts." I suggested they talk to a major bra manufacturer and obtain their methods of fitting women for bras.

The community had set a priority of collecting data on similar body shape changes happening to multiple demographics within the AIDS community. These changes included loss of fat in the face and buttocks and gaining fat in the belly and sometimes in the back of the neck. The AACTG complications RAC noted that the NIH was preparing to launch a major multi-site research study called FRAM or The Study of Fat Redistribution and Metabolic Change in HIV infection. For the AACTG to develop a competing study would be redundant and would not be the best use of limited funding.

I mention the above examples to show the careful way the committee considered all the research proposals and selected only those most likely to contribute new information on treatment for the most pressing issues of the time. The process was not easy. Within the CAB, we had heated discussions about what should be our top priorities. Many individuals were mainly concerned about issues that affected them directly. Others tried to look at the entire HIV/AIDS community rather than as separate groups by demographics or disease types. The priorities, though, were settled on by group consensus, and not by the person who spoke the loudest.

Once the priorities were finalized, each CAB representative was expected to rely on these set priorities as they voted within their respective RACs and protocol committees. The situation was similar at the AACTG committee levels. Each researcher spoke loudly in favor of research they were interested in working on. At my RAC, the chair would always ask me to share the CAB's priorities. On several occasions, the CAB priorities helped settle conflicts between competing research proposals. Ultimately, the group consensus set the research priorities for the RAC. The process was not perfect, but it helped us achieve our goals. It ensured that our resources were being used wisely and for the maximum benefit to people living with HIV and AIDS.

Off label use research. Some of the research we did in the AACTG, while I was a member, involved off label uses of approved drugs. People living with AIDS do not die of AIDS. They die of diseases that are usually rare but show up in people who no longer have a strong enough immune system to fight them. There were several situations when researchers believed that a drug approved for one disease condition might also help with a previously rare disease now becoming common in the AIDS population. I suffered from several bouts of a type of pneumonia called PCP (pneumocystis pneumonia) that is extremely rare except in people with suppressed immune systems. Insurance companies often do not want to pay for treatment that is done off label. Drug companies are reluctant to pay the millions of dollars to prove that the drug can work on the rare condition, because there isn't enough market for the use of the drug for the drug company to recoup these costs. The research must be done, though, for the FDA to approve changing the label of the drug to include the new use. If the drug has been around long enough that cheaper generic versions are available, then no one will make any money to offset the costs of the research needed to add the new use to the drug label. Federally funded research, like the research done by the AACTG, took the costs of this research away from the drug companies and used government funds to pay for the research.

Advantages of public funding. With the move toward using multiple drugs to control HIV, there was a need to find out which combinations would work better with fewer side effects. Often, research needed to be done on drugs that were manufactured by different drug companies. The AACTG, with federal funds, could help the drug companies work together to develop this research. Similarly, sometimes a drug company had a new drug that they believed might be better than a drug currently being used. To prove this, they had to set up a study comparing one group of participants who got the approved drug with another group that got the new drug. The company who made the approved drug was usually reluctant to provide their drug for a study that might prove another drug worked better. The federally funded AACTG could sponsor the study and use its funds to cover the costs of the approved drug.

Informed consent form readability. Once I got assigned to research study development groups, I let the groups know that I had a degree and work experience in news writing. News writing requires an ability to organize information so that it is more easily understood and retained. It also requires skill in editing for readability. Each group asked me to do the final edit on the informed consent forms for the research studies in development.

Many factors go into readability. I looked at the language used in the informed consent. Were the words used understandable to people who were not lawyers or medical professionals? My criteria for whether it was lay language was asking myself if I could use that word or phrase with my neighbor or someone at the grocery store without using any additional definitions.

I looked at the length of sentences. Could they be divided into smaller sentences? I looked at the length of paragraphs. Sometimes a paragraph break gives the reader's brain a chance to breathe.

I looked for long lists of items within one sentence. "The risks of the drug include nausea, diarrhea, headache, vomiting, increased blood pressure, abnormal liver function test results, and irregular heartbeat, which could be life threatening" presents information so that it is harder to understand and retain.

Using bullet points can fix this. "The risks of the drug include:

- Nausea
- Diarrhea
- Headache
- Increased blood pressure
- Abnormal liver function test results
- Irregular heartbeat, which could be life threatening"

The use of bullet points makes each risk stand out. The potentially life-threatening risk of irregular heartbeat is no longer buried at the end of a long boring sentence.

I looked at grammar and usage. Sometimes bad grammar or usage can change the meaning of a sentence.

"After taking the drug for three weeks, the doctor will examine you for any bad effects." Did the doctor take the drug for three weeks? That is what the sentence says.

"After you take the drug for three weeks, the doctor will examine you for any bad effects" is clearer. You take the drug and then the doctor examines you.

I looked for language that might trigger negative emotions. One consent form told the participants who were living with HIV that their results would be compared to the results from normal patients. This was at a time when AIDS advocates were fighting against terms like "AIDS victim" and "infected with AIDS." I believed the original language in the consent form implied that people living with HIV were not normal. "Normal" is also an ambiguous term, which could be misinterpreted. AIDS was most prevalent among gay men, people of color, and drug users. Did the writers of the consent form mean that we were not normal? Did they intend to imply that testing HIV positive meant we were not normal? I had the team change the wording from "normal patients" to "people who are HIV-negative."

"If you have been told you have sickle cell anemia, you may have more severe side effects from this drug." What if you have sickle cell anemia and it has not yet been diagnosed? Will the side effects be less severe? Will you have more side effects that are severe, or will the side effects be more severe? "If you have sickle cell anemia your side effects may be more severe" is clearer.

Lawyers and medical professionals love to use passive voice. "Blood will be drawn from you" uses passive voice. "A member of the study team will draw blood from you" is active voice. Not only is this clearer, it also forces the writer to identify who will draw the blood.

"You will be reimbursed for the costs of any unexpected harms that result from your participation in this study." Who will reimburse you? The use of passive voice allows the consent writer to leave this language vague. If you were injured by the research study, and had extra costs to treat those injuries, the doctor could say "I'm not going to reimburse you." The clinic could say "We are not going to reimburse you." The sponsor could say the same. "You will be reimbursed" does not obligate any one person or entity to take care of the reimbursement.

"The study sponsor will reimburse you for any costs directly related to harms to you that result from your participation in the study" is much clearer and obligates the sponsor to pay.

As a community advocate, I wanted to make sure the consent form could not be used against a participant who needed help. I made sure the language in the informed consent form was clear and specific.

Sometimes an early draft of a consent form will include a statement that by signing the consent form, the participant verifies that they <u>understand</u> certain risks and expectations of the study. However, there is usually no way to prove that. The participant doesn't know what they don't know. They may think they understand but may not know about relevant information that they missed when reading the consent form.

If the participant is injured in the course of a study, the sponsor could use the signed statement that includes "I understand..." against the patient. They could state: "Your signature here indicates you knew that was a risk of the study." I did my best to make sure language like this did not get included in the consent forms I reviewed.

Other community activism. The AIDS community was and is involved in medical research outside the AACTG. There are groups that meet with drug companies to advise on new AIDS research in planning. There are groups that advocate for more reasonable pricing of drugs, especially those drugs that use federal funds (taxpayer money) to cover costs of research and development. There are groups that evaluate new research on AIDS treatments and provide regular updates to people living with AIDS on the research that is enrolling new participants.

I was briefly involved in a group called AIDS Treatment Activists Coalition, or ATAC. At one meeting I attended, we advised a company that was developing new treatments for HCV. The company wanted to exclude participants of African descent because there seems to be a genetic component in this population that hinders a positive response to HCV treatment. The ATAC members reminded the company of federal guidelines against this kind of exclusion. If African Americans were not included in the research, then if the drug got approved the medical community would not know how to treat this population safely. The drug company was afraid that poor results from African Americans in the study could affect the overall study results, making it harder to get FDA approval. The ATAC members suggested using a method called stratification, showing how each demographic group responded to the new drug.

The early AIDS research activists were instrumental in changes to the FDA regulations for women in research. Traditionally, any women who were able to conceive children were banned from taking part in research if there was no proof that the study drug would not harm the developing fetus. This left a large gap in knowledge about the drug and how it would work in women and deprived these women from access to a new drug that might save or prolong their lives. Thanks to AIDS activists and others, the FDA now requires these women be included in research if they agree to use appropriate methods to prevent pregnancy.

- *Better training is needed for everyone involved in research, including the clinic staff, the researchers, the residents, the sponsors, and the sponsor monitors.*
- *Extra work is often created when research is driven by profit and not by health priorities.*
- *Economics and finance impact the conduct of research.*
- *Improvements could be made if stakeholders are willing to change and find more efficient ways of running the research program.*

From community advocate to clinic employee.

During my third year as a representative to the AACTG CAB, the director of the UAB AIDS research clinic called me into his office. He told me the clinic's regulatory coordinator had just been fired. The regulatory coordinator maintained the study records of sponsor correspondence, current protocols and consent forms, all amendments, and all IRB correspondence and approval. He evidently had not been doing his job for several months. His office was filled with stacks of paperwork, each over four feet tall, that had not been processed. There was a narrow path through the stacks to get from the office door to the desk.

The director knew about my work as the local CAB chair and as a representative to the AACTG CAB. He said the regulatory coordinator position required the same skills and knowledge that I was already using with the local and national CABs. He asked me if I would volunteer to keep the regulatory office running until he could hire a full-time replacement for the person who had been fired.

My health was improving, thanks to my new combination therapy of AIDS treatment drugs. I had been wondering if I might be well enough to return to work after twelve years on disability. I told the director I would help in the office and would try to stick to a regular eight-hour workday, to see if my stamina would hold up. As long as I was a volunteer, and not getting paid, I could still receive my disability payments from Social Security and from UAB, and would still have health insurance from Medicare, with the UAB health insurance to cover things like drug costs that were not covered by Medicare. By taking on the regulatory job as a volunteer, I could find out if I was well enough to work without losing my safety net.

Training myself. My first day in the office I realized I was going to have to train myself on how to do the regulatory job. There were no instructions. There was no handbook on what to do with the mountains of unprocessed paperwork. There was no course I could take on how to perform the daily duties of a regulatory coordinator. The IRB required me to take a course from CITI (Collaborative Institutional Training Initiative). The course gave valuable information on the history of human subjects protections, how and why research regulations evolved, and the ethical considerations. But there was nothing in the course that would help me figure out what to do with the paperwork in front of me.

I saw that there were a set of regulatory binders for each study. I noticed that there were two kinds of binders. Some were slickly produced binders that came from the drug company sponsors. These section tabs in these binders were provided with the binder and were numbered in the order that the sponsor wanted them. Each section had instructions for what needed to go into that section. I noticed some of the tabbed sections were empty except for a note to file that said the contents of that section were stored with the study coordinator or in the drug information files in the clinic's storage room. These binders were designed for clinics that only had one employee in charge of the study records. Since our clinic had divided the labor, the master binders were in my office. If sections from the binder were with the research coordinator or the data manager, a note to file was added to the master files in my office to verify the location of these records.

The other binders were less "slick" and had locally made graphics for the spine and handwritten tabs. These were for the AACTG studies and for the investigator-initiated studies (research not sponsored by a drug or device company, and usually limited to participants at UAB). I assumed that if there was a local format for keeping records then one of these binders would show that. It turned out the sections in these binders were not significantly different than the sections in the binders for industry sponsored studies.

I picked a study and went through the regulatory binders for that study, looking at how the information was organized, any cover letters or date stamps on each document, what documents were collected, etc. There was a section for the protocol documents. The most recent version of the protocol was on top, with previous versions in chronological order behind it. On top of each protocol was a copy of the approval letter from the IRB for that version of the protocol. Another section contained the consent forms, again in chronological order, with the most recent version on top, and with the IRB approval letter for each version of the consent form on top of that version. Each consent form in the folder also had an IRB approval stamp on it, showing the approval date. There was a section for sponsor correspondence. It contained letters and emails from the sponsor. Many of these were cover letters that came with new protocol versions, new consent form, or new information on the study drugs. Each letter had instructions for what to do with the documents. The instructions might require a signature from the principal investigator (PI), a submission to the IRB, a reply to the sponsor to verify that the information was received, and/or a deadline for the IRB approval and/or the PI signature. I looked around the office at the stacks of unprocessed documents. I realized I needed to find everything with a deadline and set a priority for getting these documents processed and the responses back to the sponsor.

The sponsor correspondence included cover letters for product information like revised investigator brochures for the study drugs. I could not find where these investigator brochures were filed. They were not in my office. I found out that they were in a storage room down the hall, and were sorted by the drug, not by the study. This seemed complicated to me. Like the regulatory binders in my office, each study drug document was accompanied by an IRB approval letter. If the same drug was used in multiple studies, there might be a stack of IRB approval letters, because the new document had to be submitted to the IRB for each applicable study.

There was a section in the regulatory binder for IRB correspondence. A lot of this correspondence was emails notifying the study teams of upcoming deadlines for submission of continuing review paperwork to the IRB. From the CITI training, I knew that each expedited and full Board review study had to have continuing review and IRB approval renewal at least once a year. I looked at the stacks of paperwork in the office and wondered how many of our studies were no longer IRB approved because of missed deadlines. The answer came later that day. The administrative assistant for the research clinic brought me an urgent letter from the IRB. It said that our research clinic was frozen until all research studies were brought up to date. That meant we could not open any new studies, or enroll any new patients in current studies, until the IRB lifted the freeze. Another requirement for lifting the freeze was that every member of every study team had to re-take the CITI course. I had my work cut out for me.

Cleaning up the mess. The clinic had a large conference room with enough tables for all the clinic staff (research clinic and outpatient clinic) to meet for lunch each Friday. I asked the administrative assistant if I could use the room for a few days. I set up each table in the room with a sign saying what kind of document would go on that table. One table was for protocol amendments. Another was for revised consent forms. Several tables were for information on study drugs, with a table for each of the drugs. I borrowed a cart, moved all the mountains of documents out of my office and into the conference room, and started sorting. Once I had everything sorted by type, I went into each table and sorted each in chronological order. I used sticky notes to identify anything with a missed deadline. These would get first priority for processing.

I took all the sorted documents back to my office and started work on anything that needed to go to the IRB. This seemed to be the most urgent task, to meet the IRB requirements for lifting the hold on new studies and new enrollment. I saw in the binders that the IRB had forms I needed to use for the IRB submissions. There were no instructions on how to find the forms. I located the IRB web site on my computer. I found the forms there. Each had bare minimum instructions on how to fill out the form and how to get it to the IRB office. There were a lot of terms I did not understand. I looked them up in the dictionary, only to discover that the IRB was using the terms differently than the dictionary definition. I had to ask colleagues and IRB staff to find out the IRB definitions. I wished again for training or other resources on how to do this work. I had figured out a lot on my own, but I wondered if I had figured it out correctly. One of the research coordinators told me that monitors, from the sponsors, came by the site regularly to make sure the files were in order. She suggested the monitors might help to train me when they came.

After I was well into the process of sorting and processing the documents in the office, the research clinic director offered me the job full time. I had become personally invested in making the records right and was unwilling to let anyone else come in who might let my work go to waste. But I also knew I had a good income from disability, and that as long as I had disability from UAB I would also have good health insurance. It was a difficult decision to make but I felt like a door was opening. I accepted the job, becoming a full-time employee of the research clinic.

Research priorities and capitalism. As I sorted through the documents and began processing them, I noticed a major difference between the research for the clinic and research within the AACTG. At the AACTG level, priorities were set before research could be developed and started. The resources went to fill a pre-specified need. At the clinic, I realized that there did not seem to be the same process for determining priorities for the industry-sponsored studies.

The priority for the drug companies seemed geared more to the possibility of profit from a drug. We were conducting several studies for drugs that were minimally different from drugs that were already approved. The market for this type of drug had been established. Other companies wanted a "piece of the pie," developing drugs that only differed in minor ways, such as a reduced side effect or reduced risks. With the right marketing, the company making the new drug could realize a big profit.

The people living with AIDS may not have needed this "me too" drug as much as they needed a new class of drugs. A new class of drugs would open the door for better treatment for patients whose virus was resistant to the current drugs. "Me too" drugs didn't usually help with this. If a patient had virus that was resistant to one nucleoside reverse transcriptase inhibitor, the virus would likely be resistant to most "new and improved" NRTI drugs that were designed to compete with currently approved NRTIs.

Why did the clinic do these "me too" studies? They brought in money. This money could be used to buy new equipment, pay for new staff members, and cover the losses from studies that did not bring in additional revenue. The AACTG studies did offer some payment to the clinic to cover costs but the payment was not enough. We lost money on every patient we enrolled in these studies. The industry sponsored studies helped offset that.

We had studies that were trying to prove that an older drug, already approved for medical uses outside of HIV, could be useful in treatment of AIDS or AIDS-related illness or side effects. If the manufacturer was sponsoring the study, they probably saw a chance to make more money off a product that may have peaked in sales for the initial use it was approved for.

Drugs that were approved for leprosy might help treat AIDS

related pneumonia. Anti-nausea drugs that were designed for use in pregnant women were taken off the market because of side effects in the developing fetus. Could these drugs be safely used for nausea side effects from HIV medicines if the women in the study used birth control? If there was a chance that the drug could be useful enough to make money for the sponsor, the sponsor needed this research in order to petition the FDA for a new "indication" for the drug. This means the drug would be FDA approved for the treatment in HIV patients and insurance would cover the drug.

Protecting patients from researchers. For some groups of patients, the UAB 1917 Clinic (the outpatient clinic treating HIV and AIDS patients) had to set some priorities for research projects. For instance, there was a special research interest for patients who came to the clinic during the seroconversion period of the HIV infection. This is the period when the patient's body starts to develop immune responses to the virus. The symptoms are like a severe case of the flu. The HIV clinic would find many of these patients by testing for HIV in the emergency room if someone came in for treatment of severe flu-like symptoms.

Some virologists thought that the seroconversion period might be a key time when the body's own immune system could be boosted enough to stop the HIV infection. Various methods were being tried. Researchers for each of these methods wanted to enroll seroconverting patients in their studies. We had other researchers who were interested in getting blood samples from these patients to use in the lab to study what happens to the immune system during the seroconversion. Epidemiologists and public health specialists wanted to interview the patients to try and trace how and when they contracted the virus. Seroconversion sometimes happened weeks or months after the initial exposure.

These patients were stressed. They thought they had the flu and were instead finding out they had HIV. Because I had survived HIV for a few years, and worked in the clinic, I was often called into the patient's room to talk with them about my experience, and let them know that an HIV diagnosis was not necessarily a death sentence. I could see that a major factor in their stress, in addition to learning that they had HIV, was the large number of researchers who wanted to use their information and blood samples. As one patient put it, "it's like everybody in this building wants a piece of me."

The outpatient clinic director noticed this, too. He led an effort to prioritize the research by scientific merit and by time restrictions. The interviews about transmission could wait. The blood samples to analyze the process of seroconversion had to be taken while the patient was still in that period. Researchers were told to find a way to ease the stress on the patients. This included doing one blood draw and asking researchers to share it. For studies that involved treatment, the clinic prioritized the ones that seemed the most promising. Since these patients were rare, data from the patients was pooled with data from other clinics to help find statistical significance.

Research for professional advancement. UAB hospital is a teaching hospital. In addition to having a medical school, we also had a large residency program to help medical school graduates from around the country continue their medical education. The HIV research clinic had many residents. The residents were required to do research as part of their residency. Many of the residents did research by reviewing patient charts from our research database.

The clinic's medical education mentors created a database committee. One of the functions of that committee was to set priorities for questions that might be answered by researching our patient data. When residents came up with research ideas, these would have to be evaluated by the database committee not only for scientific merit, but also for how well the research fit into our priorities. The main goal of these studies was to fulfill research requirements for the residency program.

The database committee ensured that these research projects also met the clinic's needs for answering questions to help improve patient care. However, there was little training for these residents on how to do the regulatory part of the research. As I became known as the "IRB guru" for the clinic, many residents came to me for help in writing their protocols and filling out their IRB submission paperwork. I wanted to help but I already had a fulltime job handling the major clinical research done by the clinic faculty physicians. When a resident came to me for help, I had to ask if they needed me for more than ten minutes. Anything beyond that would have to be approved by my manager. I wanted to help but my hands were tied. There were no courses or educational resources to help these residents.

Research from other departments. As a patient at the clinic, I knew there was other research going on in the clinic in addition to the studies that were represented by binders in my office. Some of these were the resident studies. Others were studies from other clinics and departments, like the AIDS vaccine clinic, the AIDS Prevention Trials Network, the School of Public Health, the School of Nursing, and others. UAB is part of a network called the Centers for AIDS

Research or CFAR. CFAR welcomed research from all over the UAB campus. Since these projects were not sponsored by the AIDS research clinic, I was not responsible for the regulatory records for most of them. The outpatient clinic director had to approve any of these studies before the study teams could conduct the research with the AIDS clinic patients. Not every proposal got approved. Proposals were weighed for scientific merit and for whether the results could have a direct or indirect impact on patient care. The director's decisions ensured that our clinic was not overwhelmed with too many competing studies happening at the same time.

Sponsor monitors. When the monitors for the multi-site trials came, I realized they were not going to be much help in my training. They had checklists to make sure I had everything filed and processed correctly but could offer me little training in how to file and how to make IRB submissions. I learned by finding out what had been done wrong rather than being taught how to do it right.

The first monitor I met walked into my office and announced she had a terrible hangover and asked where she could get some strong coffee. I should have sent her away and told her to come back when she was feeling better. I was new. She was my first monitor visit. I got her some coffee from the clinic break room. She opened her tablet and started going through her checklist. There were still mountains of documents filling my office. At least now they were organized by document type and deadline date. The monitor opened my binder and looked at her checklist. She asked why I hadn't filed certain documents like protocol amendments, recent approved consent forms, IRB correspondence, investigator brochures. I waved my hands over the stack of documents and explained the situation I had inherited. I tried to explain my plan for getting everything into place. She yelled at me and threatened to have our research site shut down. I told her the IRB had already done that and explained our plan for reopening with the IRB. She yelled some more. I asked her to go through the binders and send me a list of everything that was missing. As I got caught up, I could let her know which items could not be found, so she could send them again. She said she needed a drink and told me that I was asking too much from her. When she started yelling again, I stood up and told her to leave my office. Luckily, this was the worst monitor visit I had while working there. She never came back. After I told my manager what had happened, my manager called the company and demanded a different monitor for future visits. But there were plenty of other bad experiences with study monitors.

Some of the sponsor monitors worked directly for the sponsor. For instance, if the study was sponsored by Merck, then the monitor was a Merck employee. These monitors, who reported directly to the sponsor, were the most helpful. One showed me why it was important to change our drug information files so that they were organized by study, and not by drug. She also helped me figure out a system to efficiently make this change. She gave me valuable tips to better organize my records and always provided a list of items that needed attention before her next visit. Other monitors were not so helpful, especially if they worked for a Contract Research Organization or CRO.

CROs are companies that oversee research studies on behalf of sponsors. If a sponsor uses a CRO, that means the sponsor has outsourced the work of overseeing the activities of the research sites. Their monitors reported up the chain of command within the CRO, and not directly to the sponsor.

As I became more adept at my job as regulatory coordinator, I studied each protocol, comparing the protocol with the language in the consent forms and the schedule of events for the study participants. I often realized that I had a more complete understanding of the required conduct of the study than the monitor did. I also wondered if the training provided to the study monitors was adequate.

We had one monitor who was new to her company and new to living in the United States. Like most monitors, she had a checklist that she used to make sure her visits were completed thoroughly. One of the items on her checklist required her to see the CLIA waiver for our site's lab.

What is CLIA? From the CMS website: "The Centers for Medicare & Medicaid Services (CMS) regulates all laboratory testing (except research) performed on humans in the U.S. through the Clinical Laboratory Improvement Amendments (CLIA). In total, CLIA covers approximately 260,000 laboratory entities. The Division of Clinical Laboratory Improvement & Quality, within the Quality, Safety & Oversight Group, under the Center for Clinical Standards and Quality (CCSQ) has the responsibility for implementing the CLIA Program."

The objective of the CLIA program is to ensure quality laboratory testing. Although all clinical laboratories must be properly certified to receive Medicare or Medicaid payments, CLIA has no direct Medicare or Medicaid program responsibilities. If a lab was not CLIA certified, CMS could issue a waiver for the lab to conduct certain tests, such as a urine pregnancy test.

Our lab was CLIA certified, so we did not need, or have, a CLIA waiver for the lab. The monitor went to everyone on the study team asking for the waiver: the clinic director, the research director, the clinical research coordinator, the data manager, and me. She pronounced "waiver" as "way-were" because of her accent, making the discussions with clinic personnel more complicated because we didn't understand what she was looking for. After a few minutes of confusion, though, each person she asked told her we didn't have a waiver. We didn't need a waiver. We showed her our CLIA certification. There was no place on her checklist for her to indicate that our lab was certified.

For the next five years, while I was working in that office, every six months or so I would get a call or email from someone at her CRO, saying they were doing an internal audit and realized our file did not have a copy of our CLIA waiver.

Another CRO monitor was someone I had met socially but did not know well. He stepped into my office and, after we shook hands, he reached over and stroked my beard with his hand, saying he thought the beard looked great on me. I told him he did not have permission to touch my face. I reported him to my manager, who reported his actions to his supervisors at the CRO. We were assigned a different monitor.

A monitor from a smaller CRO had been friendly, but always projected a feeling of dissatisfaction with his work. After the study was completed, he made a close-out visit to our site, collecting originals of many of the study documents from our local research files. Luckily, we kept copies of the documents. About a week after his close-out visit, a manager at the CRO called to ask if we could send all the documents again. She said she would send me a list. I told her the monitor had collected all these already. She told me he had vanished. He was not answering his phone and had changed his flight back to the home office to an unknown destination. She said as far as she knew, all our study records had been dumped in a trash bin at the Dallas airport, where he was changing flights.

Monitors sometimes asked me to provide documents that were not related to the protocol or the study procedures. CROs bid for the contracts to conduct studies for major industry sponsors. Sometimes their bid includes a promise to collect even more information than is required in the federal regulations. When situations arose where the monitors asked us to do unnecessary work to make their files look better, our director would ask the monitor to show him where that was required in the Federal regulations. He said if the CRO could not show us a regulation that required it, we would not do the extra paperwork.

Informed Consent Form readability. I was often surprised at the lack of readability of the informed consent forms I got from industry sponsors. The forms were written by scientists and lawyers, with little attention paid to whether an average person could understand them. I borrowed a medical dictionary from one of the research coordinators so that I could look up lay definitions for complex medical terms used and edit these into the consent form. One time I was working on an informed consent form for a new drug that would fight the AIDS virus at a completely different part of its life cycle. The approved drugs all interrupted viral replication within the cells in the patient's body. This new drug blocked the virus from entering cells, by creating barriers to the receptors the virus used to make a path to enter the cell. The virus needed to enter the immune cell to replicate itself, so a barrier to cell entry would effectively slow down the replication of the virus.

Every investigational drug must have an FDA approved Investigator Brochure. These contain highly scientific complex language that only an advanced researcher can fully understand. The sponsor for the new drug moved two pages from the background section of the Investigator Brochure and copied the complex language, word for word, into the informed consent form for study participants.

I knew it would be impossible for our patients to understand what this language meant. Most doctors would have trouble with the language used in the brochure. The frustration of trying to read this section could easily cause a prospective participant to give up on reading the informed consent form. I deleted the two pages from the Investigator Brochure and replaced them with something like this: "The study drug fights the virus differently from other medications for treating HIV and AIDS. The study drug prevents the virus from entering the cells in your body. This helps stop the virus from growing in your body. If you would like more information, please ask your study doctor."

The sponsor did not like the changes. After some discussion, though, they agreed that I could send the track changes version to the IRB so the IRB could see the original language and my changes to the language. The IRB agreed with my changes.

When I sent a study package, amendment package, or continuing review package to the IRB, my name was on that package. My personal integrity was represented by the quality of work in the submission. I would not send something to the IRB unless I believed it was complete, accurate, and ready for approval. Monitors and sponsors often argued with me about my edits to the consent forms to make them more readable. I asked them if my edits had changed the meaning of the form. They said no, but the IRB needed to make the edits, not me. I told them the IRB expected me to prepare the submission documents so that they were as close to approvable as possible. The sponsor monitors wanted to see this in writing from the IRB. Even though I had a degree that proved my training in editing for readability, and considerable experience doing it, the sponsors wanted me to just shuffle the paperwork on to the IRB with as few changes as possible.

<u>Teaching the sponsor and CRO.</u> While I was working at the AIDS research clinic, HIPAA (Health Insurance Portability and Accountability ACT) went into effect. HIPAA was primarily designed to allow sharing of medical records so that health insurance records would not be lost if you changed jobs or changed insurance companies. A major impact of HIPAA was that the medical record information be kept confidential to the greatest extent possible. A patient had to sign a HIPAA authorization form to allow their protected health information (PHI) to be shared. This requirement extended to research activities.

About the same time that HIPAA went into effect, drug manufacturers felt the need to collect information on what impact an experimental drug might have on pregnancy and/or a developing fetus. Ethical considerations would not allow researchers to give drugs with unknown side effects to pregnant women. The risks would be too great. Because of these risks, study participants had to agree to prevent pregnancy for themselves, if they were female, or with their female partner, if the study participant was male. Drug companies knew that sometimes, even with the best intentions and the best available contraceptive methods, pregnancies can happen. They started adding language to informed consent forms stating that they wanted to collect data on any such pregnancy that did occur. Because of the new HIPAA requirements, most sponsors developed a separate consent form for pregnant partners of male participants. The pregnant partners would have to agree and sign the consent form before any data on the pregnancy or fetus could be collected.

One drug company sent me an amendment to a study that was currently open at our site. The amendment added the information about collecting pregnant partner data to the study protocol. The sponsor's template consent was edited to add that "if you are male, and your female partner should become pregnant while you are on the study, we will ask you to tell us if there are any problems with the pregnancy or with the baby when it is born."

In the United States, there are few if any instances where a man could give information about his female partner's health without her written permission. I told the sponsor this and refused to send the consent changes to the IRB until the language was changed to "if you are male, and your female partner should become pregnant while you are on the study, we will ask her to give permission for us to follow the pregnancy and its outcomes." I also told the sponsor they would need to provide a consent form for the pregnant partner to sign. The sponsor refused to make the changes. We were at an impasse.

The amendment included major changes to the study design and new risk information on the study drugs that the participants needed to know about. Because of this, I reluctantly agreed to send the submission to the IRB. I made notes within the submission that I didn't think the pregnant partner information was approvable as it was written. The IRB agreed. The final decision was that the IRB approved everything else in the amendment except the addition of data collection from pregnant partners.

The study eventually completed and closed at our site. We never collected any information on the pregnant partners for this study. I was flabbergasted that the leadership team at the sponsor's CRO had so little understanding of the HIPAA privacy laws. As a study team member for other studies, I had been required to have extensive training from each of our sponsors, and from UAB, on the HIPAA law. It was evident that the leaders at the CRO did not have the same training requirements.

Most of the studies I worked on were sponsored by the AACTG. As a major player in AIDS research, with NIH funding, they could demand and get only the best and most experienced monitors for their studies. One of the AACTG monitors would joke with me that they should hire me to go ACTG sites and teach people how to maintain research regulatory files. I told him that I had taught myself, with a little help from monitors, the IRB staff, and the research clinic director. I suggested that even if it wasn't me, the research at other sites would benefit from having someone do regulatory training, so others wouldn't have to learn the hard way like I did.

Financial disclosures and conflicts of interest.

Money has always been an issue in medical research. This became more evident in 1999 after a participant in a clinical trial died. The clinical trial was tainted by financial conflicts of interest. A young man named Jesse Gelsinger had a rare genetic condition that caused a metabolic disorder. The condition could be treated. The standard treatment was extensive and not always successful. Gelsinger was offered the chance to participate in a clinical trial of a genetic therapy that could help with his condition. When he was tested for eligibility just before starting the treatment, the tests showed that he was not well enough for the treatment.

He should have been excluded from the study. The hospital and some of the study doctors had significant financial interests in the outcome of the study. Because they needed to enroll patients to keep the research going, they allowed Gelsinger to receive the experimental treatment. His body could not handle the impact of the treatment, and he died shortly after receiving it.

The government responded quickly. Soon every investigator on any study team had to disclose financial interests in companies involved with the research studies. Institutions set up Conflict of Interest Review Boards (CIRBs). The CIRBs worked with the IRBs to ensure that financial considerations would not impact the ethical conduct of research. Investigators with significant financial interests, such as being a major stockholder, might have to withdraw from a study team, or might not be allowed to take part in the selection of participants or in the informed consent process. Any significant financial interests had to be disclosed in the informed consent form, so that potential study participants could decide for themselves if they could trust the study team to have their best interests in mind. While this was a start, only limiting the disclosures to financial interests meant that other factors were not disclosed. Factors like needing to complete a research study in order to get tenure, needing to complete a research study in order to complete requirements for an advanced degree, or wanting the professional boost for being an author on a publication in a respected journal can potentially bias study team members. However, this information is not collected, or formally reported to participants or to the IRB.

In some cases, the effects of financial interests could be more subtle. The AIDS research clinic at UAB is one of the top AIDS research clinics in the world. The clinic director, and several of the other investigators, are experts in various aspects of treating HIV and AIDS, and in how to develop better treatments. Drug companies seek out experts like the UAB physicians to consult in investigational drug development, and to speak at stockholder meetings to explain AIDS treatments and how they work. The money these physicians earn from these activities with industry sponsors often goes above the threshold at which reporting is required. Our director always included a statement in his financial disclosure report that this financial interest could not bias him in favor of that sponsor or that drug, because he did the same consulting and speaking work for almost every company that developed drugs to treat HIV and AIDS.

I never saw any evidence where a participant was put in danger because of the financial involvement our physicians had with drug companies. What I did see, though, was our site opening a lot of studies of "me too" drugs because our physicians had consulted on the development of the research studies for these experimental drugs. The studies offered little new treatment beyond what was already available by prescription or in other research studies we were doing. Often the "me too" studies opened and completed before any participants ever enrolled at UAB. For me, this proved that there was no bias in the physicians that would have caused them to enroll a participant in a study inappropriately.

The major harm, if you can call it that, was that these extra research studies created significant extra work for the clinic staff, including me. None of us had time to spare for these projects. We wished that we could concentrate on the research that offered real benefits to the patients in our clinic, rather than helping to bring copycat drugs into the market to boost the profits for a drug manufacturer. These research studies meant extra work for the IRB and the IRB staff, too. When I would run into the IRB chairman on campus, he would always say "your clinic needs to concentrate on studies that will enroll a lot of patients, and quit doing these studies that don't enroll anyone or only enroll one or two."

What none of us considered is that each of the investigational "me too" drugs might have a subtle difference that reduced a major side effect, or that would allow the drug to work against the HIV even if the virus had developed resistance to similar drugs in the same class. For one or two patients, the drug could be a life saver. Maybe the extra work to open and run a "me too" study was worth it if a life could be saved. If the study provided the drug at no cost to participants, having a "me too" study could help a patient who could not afford the similar approved drugs.

Other economic and financial impacts. Finances affect research in other ways. While I was working in the HIV clinic, research at the entire university got temporarily shut down because a former employee of the grants and contracts office charged that some research was billing both the study sponsor and the participant's insurance for the same procedure. This is called double billing. The aftermath of the charge and the investigation was that UAB had to create a separate department to review billing plans on research projects and approve these plans. The new billing compliance office worked with the clinics and the grants and contracts office to ensure that double billing would not happen.

Research jobs in hospital and academic research centers usually pay less than jobs with CROs. While I was working in the HIV research clinic, we lost a few research team members who were hired away by CROs offering much higher salaries. Training of new employees is costly. Some of us wondered if the University could avoid the costs of continually training new employees by offering the current employees a salary that would compete with what the CROs were offering.

Conducting research on a new drug is a costly venture for drug companies. Sometimes the research results indicate that the company is not going to be able to sell enough product to offset the costs. When that happens, companies often get creative in how to boost projected sales. Several times study sponsors would add a quality of life survey to their study design after the study had been running for some time. I assumed they were hoping the survey might show a difference in how the participants felt, even if the data collected did not show any difference in medical outcomes between the study drug and the approved drug used for comparison.

Once, after a study was completed, the sponsor asked us to let them conduct a quality of life study, including surveys, interviews, and focus groups, on the former participants of the study. This was after the study results failed to show the anticipated reduction of side effects when compared with the drug that was currently used in standard practice. We did not allow the company to do this, because they wanted to do it independently of our clinic staff. We would have no oversight but would be liable if anything went wrong.

Finding more efficient ways to work. After I had been in my job for a few months, I got asked to design a research protocol for the AIDS research clinic. The clinic was developing an electronic database of all our research records. The goal was to combine our data with other sites in the Centers for AIDS Research (CFAR). Work was already underway to standardize terminology and records keeping across the CFAR sites to make this collaboration possible. Our clinic director felt that if we were using the database for research and sharing the data with other clinics for collaborative research, we needed to get IRB approval for this.

Up until that time, the residents who worked on chart review research products from the database were responsible for submitting each project to the IRB for review and approval before collecting the data. I proposed that in the future, we fold all these projects into the database protocol. I would write the protocol to describe who would have access to the database for research, how the data would be collected and protected, and what kinds of research questions would be answered by the projects. At each annual continuing review, I would provide the IRB with a list of all the projects that were ongoing, and information about any publications that resulted in the past year from the database research. Each member of the database group was listed as an investigator on the project. I collected CVs and training records to send to the IRB. The IRB was open to reviewing one "blanket" protocol that was submitted by someone who knew how to do IRB submissions, instead of dozens of individual projects each year. The residents were relieved that they no longer had to do their own IRB submissions. I was able to bypass the problem that the residents did not have sufficient training in regulatory practices by finding an efficient way to combine the projects and take over the regulatory duties.

Using a central IRB. While I was working in the AIDS research clinic, the UAB IRB made a major change. A commercial IRB, called Western IRB or WIRB, was added to the list of IRBs that researchers at UAB could use for their study approval and oversight. WIRB became the required

"IRB of record" for any studies that were sponsored by drug companies or device companies. Most of the "me too" studies were industry sponsored. Sending them to WIRB took the regulatory burden for the study off the local research team and the UAB IRB. The local research team was helped because WIRB had already approved the study itself. I only had to send in paperwork about the study team and the research facilities, so that WIRB could approve the study.

Other research sites across the country felt the same relief if they sent these studies to WIRB or a similar central IRB. The UAB IRB still had to review paperwork for completeness before sending the package on to WIRB. This was much less work than handling the review and approval process locally, though. Sponsors benefitted because they only had to work with one IRB, instead of an IRB for each site. The system of using a central IRB made opening research for one or two patients at our site much less burdensome. I felt like this was a good solution for most research. If a study was controversial, or would have issues unique to our site, we could ask the local IRB to review it instead. Sometimes the local IRB made that decision for us.

Incentive to move on. Most of the time, training for an industry sponsored study would be held at a major convention center in a tourist friendly location. Only the principal investigator and the clinical research coordinator would be invited to attend. I never attended one of these trainings held in an exclusive resort. Usually the clinical research coordinator would bring me some folders and instructions but didn't remember much about the regulatory training. One sponsor, though, wanted to conduct training for the entire research staff. The CRO, one of the largest in the business, sent a team to the UAB AIDS research clinic, and conducted training for three days. Half of one day was devoted just to regulatory requirements. One statement that the trainers repeatedly made was "the IRB always has the last word." Every time I heard that statement in the training, I would think about changing jobs to work for the IRB. The IRB staff repeatedly told me that I was the best regulatory coordinator they worked with. In 2007, there was an opening at the IRB office to replace an assistant director who was retiring. I got the job!

5 RESEARCH OVERSIGHT
(INSTITUTIONAL REVIEW BOARD)

- *Many of the same problems I saw in the AIDS research clinic were amplified at the IRB level.*
- *There is little "nuts and bolts" education provided for IRB staff.*
- *Everyone involved in research, including the IRB and IRB staff, needs to have the capacity for critical thinking.*
- *Researchers, sponsors, students, mentors, and hospital administrators need more education on what IRBs do and what IRBs need to do their work.*
- *Priorities for research need to be set at the institutional level and work their way down to the individual researchers.*
- *The institution needs to provide adequate support to meet these priorities.*
- *All stakeholders need to be willing to make changes to improve research and increase efficiency.*

<u>Lack of training for IRB staff.</u> I was initially hired by the IRB for a technical writer position. This allowed me to be employed at the IRB office before retirement started for the person I was replacing. The goal was to have me train with her for three weeks. However, she met with Human Resources and found out that if she wanted to use her accumulated paid time off hours, she could effectively retire in one week. That week got reduced to three days, because she wanted time to say goodbye to the others in the office. She had worked at the IRB many years and developed some strong friendships in the office.

Even though I was familiar with the subject matter, and had

been the recipient of IRB reviews, I did not know the review process for IRB staff members. The position I was taking was assigned to work on the minimal risk studies that did not need to go to the full Board for review. No one on the IRB staff except the person I was replacing had any experience with reviewing minimal risk research. There were no online training courses or manuals to tell me what I needed to do. The IRB had policies and procedures, but the procedures were not in the same document as the policies. The procedures for minimal risk studies were vague at best. I found out that the standard process for reviewing the minimal risk studies at the UAB IRB was often different than the process described in the published policies and procedures. I tried studying the code of federal regulations but found out that UAB IRB's standard practice was more demanding than what the federal code required. I went into the files to see how my predecessor had handled situations, just as I had done when I started at the HIV clinic.

I also got help from a website called The IRB Forum. IRB staff from all over post questions and get answers. Sometimes the answers would conflict with each other. The number of questions posted told me that I was not the only IRB professional who needed more guidance.

Resistance to change and improvements. Another similarity to the HIV clinic job was that when I started, there were large stacks of unprocessed documents on my shelf and a filing cabinet filled with studies that were partially processed, waiting for the study team to respond to requests for changes. The submissions were coming in faster than one person could process them. Much of my learning was done by trial and error. I was criticized by my manager and by study teams for my slow turnaround times. When I found ways to speed up the process, the IRB chairman said I could not possibly do a complete initial review in such a short time. I slowed down again. I took work home with me and worked nights and weekends at home, going well beyond a forty-hour work week, but could not get caught up.

Sometimes I had a volunteer to help with time consuming chores like pulling files and filing documents. But if another part of the IRB office needed help, or if budget cuts required cutbacks, my helpers were always the first to go. The emphasis in the IRB office was on the studies that required full Board review. The minimal risk studies were treated like a nuisance.

Lack of training for student researchers and mentors. One reason that minimal risk studies were treated like a nuisance was that almost every department in the university required degree candidates to do a research project. These departments counted on the IRB records to prove the students had done the projects.

I reviewed research submissions from the School of Nursing, the School of Public Health, the School of Education, the School of Medicine, the School of Social Work, the Business school, and others, even the Department of Theatre and Dance. Most of these submissions, per the regulations, should have been deemed "Not Human Subjects Research" by the departments and not sent to the IRB. An education student shadowing an experienced teacher and taking notes on the teaching methods does not meet the "generalizable knowledge" criteria for Human Subjects Research. A satisfaction survey done by the medical library is quality improvement, and not generalizable. A focus group of medical students discussing whether they feel they have gotten adequate training in a field of medicine is quality improvement, and not generalizable beyond UAB. A student nurse interviewing other nurses about their perceptions of a certain procedure they must do is specific to her department, and not generalizable. But I reviewed these, usually as Expedited Review, because that is the way the UAB IRB did things at that time.

The time spent reviewing these minimal risk studies increased due to the lack of adequate training for these student and resident researchers on how to complete IRB submissions. Even though all research staff had to complete online training in research regulations and ethics, the courses offered no training on filling out IRB forms. My stack of unprocessed submission documents continued to grow while I took constant phone calls from students and residents asking me to help them.

The students, residents, and even some of the faculty researchers quickly forgot the information from the online courses in regulations and ethics. Here are some of the questions and comments I have gotten over the years, from investigators who had completed online training in research regulations.

- "It's not research, I'm just drawing blood to analyze." "Just drawing blood" does not mean a project is not research. What kind of analysis is being done? What question are you trying to answer with your analysis? Is this a systematic investigation designed to contribute to generalizable knowledge?

- "It's not research, I'm just collecting data on standard of care." Are you collecting the data in such a way that you cannot link it back to the patient's chart? What are you doing with the data? Are you using it to contribute to generalizable knowledge?

- "I need to make the study higher risk so I can get published." This is an unfortunate side effect of the requirement that that faculty members must have publications in scholarly journals to get promoted or to get tenure. However, the role of the IRB is to make sure that risks are minimized to the greatest extent possible. If you can obtain a strong comparison between drug A and drug B by looking at historical outcomes in an extensive review of patient records, then there is likely no need to expose patients to the added risks of a randomized clinical trial. If the research question requires a randomized clinical trial, do one. But if you can answer the research question with less risk, the IRB should require you to use the less risky methods. Your desire to get published should not factor into the IRB's review of the ethics of your study design.

- We paid millions for the equipment needed to do this study. You have to approve it. You would think that hospital departments would make sure the study was feasible before investing money in the equipment to do it. The hospitals I worked at did not have a system to check this. When the IRB was faced with a choice of protecting study participants or protecting the hospital budget, we had to remember that our job is protecting the participants. Because the people who approve expenses don't understand the IRB review and approval process, they did not consider the IRB review and approval process when allowing the equipment to be purchased.

- "You must review this as expedited. We need some level of IRB review for our studies so we can retain our nursing Magnet status." "Magnet status" is an award given by the American Nurses' Credentialing

Center (ANCC) to hospitals that satisfy a set of criteria designed to measure the strength and quality of their nursing. ANCC is an affiliate of the American Nurses Association. Achieving Magnet status is considered an honor for the nursing program at a hospital. It promises to help the hospital attract better nurses, especially nursing researchers. Online information about magnet status indicates that a magnet hospital's nursing department shows excellence in leadership, innovation, and patient care.

At the hospitals where I have worked, "excellence in innovation" has been interpreted as achieving a minimum number of research and publications within a set period. For a hospital where there is already a strong research component within the nursing department, this is not an issue. For a hospital that needs to create a strong research component, sometimes the need for volume supersedes the need for quality and applicability to patient care.

As with other disciplines, nurses who want to be excellent nurses, but have no desire to conduct research, sometimes feel pressured to have a research study published to achieve professional growth or job security. This pressure is heightened by the desire of nursing administration to achieve Magnet status. I believe there should be other ways to recognize nursing excellence in innovation. Certainly, many nursing research studies have improved patient care dramatically. But when pressure for volume takes over, IRBs are forced to review studies that have little or no impact on patient care, and do not help show nursing excellence. A nurse who does not want to be a researcher, but is forced to do research in order to get an advanced degree or to alleviate pressure from hospital management, will often turn to conducting surveys of nurses' perceptions of certain common practices.

The perceptions of a group of nurses at one hospital is highly unlikely to contribute to generalizable knowledge. It is not human subjects research. This does not mean the research is not important. It only means that the research probably does not need oversight by the IRB. The need for publication in a scholarly journal is not a criterion the IRB should consider when determining the review level required for a research project. Neither is the desire of the nursing program to achieve magnet status. However, many journals and conferences require a document from the IRB to verify that the IRB either approved the research or determined that the research was not subject to the IRB. I advised the nurse researchers in situations like this to use the shorter form we provided for Not Human Subjects Research and send it to the IRB so that we could issue a determination letter.

- "I don't need to learn how to do research, I just need to get a paper published." Nurses are not the only group who feels the pressure to get published. But all these groups have one thing in common. There is little training available on how to conduct research. Nursing schools and medical schools require training in statistics as part of their degree requirements. But programs that also require courses in research regulations and research regulatory process, if they exist at all, are rare. Institutions with generous funding may have a budget for a mentor or trainer on their IRB staff. In my experience, this is rare.

Some institutions have a separate department for research operations that provide training. But these training programs are usually geared for the research that brings funding into the institution. For most research that is funded, the industry sponsor takes over the training for the research team. For studies that are investigator initiated and have gotten a grant from the NIH or another funding agency, the institution's research operations or sponsored programs department handles this training. If a study is not funded, there is usually little training available. Individuals who feel forced to conduct research often have nowhere to turn for help. They hope the IRB staff can help them. Some IRB have developed self-training tools and online courses to help with this. Sadly, most IRB offices don't have the time to provide researcher training on a face to face basis.

- <u>"Why do I need to complete training? Can't you just tell me how to fill out this form?"</u> The IRB staff is not going to conduct your study for you. If you don't know enough about the regulations and policies and procedures to fill out a simple application form, how are you going to ensure that your research is conducted ethically? This is why we require training.

- <u>"The participants are nurses, we aren't collecting patient PHI, so confidentiality does not apply."</u> This is a common mistake made by investigators in medical settings. They think the regulations that protect study participants only apply if the participants are patients. Even if the participants are hospital employees, the research team must ensure that their confidentiality and privacy are protected.

- "Yes, we are using the device off label, but it's minimal risk because it's standard practice." This question points out the need for research team education. The regulations for devices differ from the regulations for drugs. A device study can only be reviewed as minimal risk/expedited review if the device is being used according to the FDA approved uses listed in the device labeling. Research involving off label use of a device is, by definition, more than minimal risk. For drugs, though, there are some instances where a research study can use a drug off label and still be considered minimal risk. Maybe this is because a drug can be easily discontinued but a device that is implanted into a patient's body cannot usually be easily removed. As an IRB manager, I saw device companies trying to get around this by saying that the study is collecting "real world" data on the use of the device, which could include off label uses. If the study is prospective, collecting data in real time, I always err on the side of caution and require full Board review if data is being collected on off label uses.

- "Why do I have to obtain informed consent?" This is a common but complex question. Usually the person asking it wants a simple answer, because they do not understand the multiple issues that must be considered. You can't give a simple answer for most questions that require critical thinking. There needs to be more education for researchers so that they can understand the issues. There are many variables that must be looked at in the study design and in the type of consent or type of waiver that is most important. Sorting through the variables requires critical thinking.

Many researchers don't want to obtain signed consent and would do anything they could to avoid this requirement. They would cite a previous study. I would have to explain why the two studies were different and had different requirements. I developed a decision tree to help explain to researchers the factors that must be considered when deciding whether to require signed informed consent. Many of the researchers I worked with could not or would not use this education tool. If they had used it, the decision tree/chart would have helped them discern if they needed to obtain signed consent, request a waiver of consent documentation, request a waiver of consent, or request a waiver of consent elements.

The decision tree asks a series of questions related to the risk level of the study, whether PHI will be collected, and whether the investigator has contact with the research subjects in order to guide the researcher toward obtaining consent, requesting a waiver of consent, requesting a waiver of consent documentation, or requesting a waiver of consent elements.

"Waiver of consent documentation" means that consent is obtained, but no signature is required. An example of this is a survey study. The researcher would ask "would you like to take part in a survey?" If the person being asked said yes, the survey would proceed. Saying "yes" conveyed consent. A signature is not needed.

"Waiver of consent" means the study design meets certain criteria that allow the IRB to waive consent. The researcher must explain why it would be difficult or impossible to conduct the research without the waiver. An example of this is a data collection of past information from patients' medical records. If the patients are no longer being seen at the clinic it would be difficult to have a consent process. The other criteria that must be met in the study design include showing that the research poses minimal risk to patients, that it could not be conducted without the protected health information (PHI) found in the medical records, and telling whether or not results will be made available once the research is completed.

"Waiver of consent elements" means the IRB determines that some of the required elements of the consent process can be left out and altered, if the study design explains why this is necessary. An example is research that requires drawing blood immediately after a severe trauma and the patient is not conscious. The IRB can alter the elements of consent to allow the blood draw, with the condition that the blood not be used if consent, from the patient or the legally authorized representative of the patient, cannot be obtained within a specified time.

The decision tree was designed as an attempt to teach the process of using critical thinking to go beyond learning regulations and definitions and start to apply these in practice. Anyone doing research needs to do this. Memorization is not enough. Critical thinking is essential. Since I could not persuade other departments at the hospital to assume the responsibility of training researchers and research team members in applying the regulations, and did not have the staff for the IRB to take on this individualized instruction, making the decision tree was the best I could do.

- **Using a consent form that is not IRB approved.** An IRB usually would not know this is happening. Most IRBs require the study team to include a copy of the current approved consent form as part of the required continuing review submission. Even so, mistakes occur. The wrong consent form might be used in a consent process. When this happens, the team is required to send a deviation report to the IRB, along with a corrective action plan describing how, in the future, they will ensure that the most recent approved consent form is always used when consenting participants.

  At one institution where I worked, the IRB had dozens of staff members. Many of them had little direct contact with research teams. Often an IRB staff member would enroll in a study for their own reasons but use their participation to provide some inside information on whether the study is being conducted properly. Once, a co-worker brought me her copy of an informed consent form she was asked to sign. The form had not yet been reviewed by the IRB, did not match anything we had on file, and did not have an IRB stamp. The basic education we required for research team members included a module on the consent process. In this case, the study team did not remember the training and did not make sure they were using the most recent approved consent form.

- **"If you want to be treated at this clinic, you have to take part in this research study."** Sometimes this is OK. Sometimes it isn't. Clinics and hospitals often let patients know that their medical data will be used for research purposes. Sometimes they allow patients to opt out. Sometimes the institution does not have the technology to allow patients to opt out. What is important is that the IRB approves the plan for using the data and that the patients are fully informed of this. Sometimes, however, clinics go beyond this. The same IRB staff member who uncovered the unapproved consent form also ran into this situation. She wanted an appointment at a pain clinic. The head of the clinic was running a study on an experimental pain treatment. The IRB staff member was told she could not receive any pain treatment, even approved pain treatment, unless she agreed to take part in the study of the experimental treatment. Not only was this unethical, but the requirement to take part in the study in order to receive any treatment was not in the protocol that the IRB reviewed and approved. The investigator was reprimanded and required to take the online ethics training again. I wondered if he would retain the information this time, since he did not retain after he first took the course.

- "I'm too busy to send you a continuing review. Can you give me an extension?" The federal requirements state that all human subjects research that is not exempt must be reviewed by the IRB at least once a year. This is called continuing review. The IRB cannot extend the expiration date for the IRB approval. If continuing review is not reviewed and approved before the set deadline, the IRB approval lapses. This is emphasized in the training that investigators must take. Most IRBs also repeat this requirement in their approval letters. If the researchers had paid attention when they took their training, they would not ask this question. If they are too busy to fill out the required paperwork, maybe they are too busy to properly conduct the research.

- "You have no idea how hard it is to do research when you are a resident." The IRB cannot change the regulations because your residency keeps you busy. Your residency mentor may be able to change your residency requirements to include time to do research, since research is a requirement for your residency program. The residency program needs to include education on time management. Maybe not every resident needs to do research.

- "I never knew we had to list students on our research team." IRBs must know the names of everyone working on a study so that the IRB can maintain training records and credentials on all research team members. Other departments ask the IRB to verify if someone worked on a study. For instance, if research work is part of a degree requirement, the school will likely ask the IRB to confirm that the student fulfilled this requirement. The IRB cannot do this unless the person is listed on the submission form sent to the IRB.

The consequences of the omission were severe for the students. I got countless calls from sobbing students saying: "They won't let me graduate." There was nothing I could do. The person who made this statement did not read the IRB application form. The IRB application form for a study specifically stated: "List all personnel involved in the study in the space below." If students are working on a study, they must be included in "all personnel." The students had relied on their faculty mentor for guidance. The faculty mentor did not know the IRB policies and procedures, the policies and requirements of the graduate school, or the regulations governing human subjects research.

- Underline: But it's the New England Journal of Medicine! A
resident at the hospital called me, begging me to give
an approval for a study he had already completed. He
had not submitted the study to the IRB in advance of
doing the research because he felt like it would be
classified as Not Human Subjects Research. Our web
site made it clear that only the IRB could make an
official NHSR determination. Our policies and
procedures did not allow us to make a retroactive
determination. The resident had presented the results
of the study at a conference. An editor from the New
England Journal of Medicine was in the audience.
After the presentation, the editor asked the resident to
submit the study to him for publication. Then he
asked if the IRB had reviewed the research. When the
resident told him "no" the editor said they could not
publish the article without an IRB approval or IRB
determination letter, verifying the IRB knew about the
research before it was done. The resident was frantic.
NEJM is one of the most prestigious medical journals.
A publication credit in the journal would ensure a
good position for the resident when his residency
completed. The best I could do was to issue a letter
stating that the IRB had not received any information
on the study prior to the research being done. The
letter added that after looking at the study design, I
had determined that if it had been sent to the IRB
prior to the research being done, I would likely have
made the determination that it was Not Human
Subjects Research and not subject to IRB oversight.
The restrictions posed by the journal, the federal
guidelines, and by the IRB's policies and procedures,
are complicated. This is why I have advocated for
more education for would-be researchers. With more
education, heartbreaking situations like this could be

avoided. The resident had relied on his faculty mentor for guidance. The faculty mentor did not know the IRB policies and procedures, or the regulations governing human subjects research.

- "The only way we can prove the concept is if we give each participant a risky procedure, even if they are not in the group that is getting treatment." One IRB I worked at was asked to review a study that was testing a potential new treatment that involved collecting stem cells from bone marrow during a spinal tap procedure and then directly injecting these stem cells into a diseased or damaged organ in the participant's body. The study had a control group, which would still have the bone marrow collection and the injection into a diseased organ, but the injection would be saline only, with no stem cells. The study team wanted to make the study blinded, so that the participants would not know if they were getting stem cells or saline placebo. Even the placebo group would have the spinal tap and bone marrow collection, and the injection of placebo (instead of stem cells) into the diseased organ, so that participants would not know which group they were in. The bone marrow collection, the spinal tap, and the stem cell (or placebo) injections were high risk procedures. The IRB correctly spent a great deal of time debating the ethics of doing "sham procedures" on participants who would have only risks and no chance of benefit. The investigator became angry at the amount of time and information the IRB needed to complete its review. IRBs are charged with verifying that research is ethical and that risks to all participants are minimized. The education and training this investigator completed made this clear. If he had retained the information from the training, he would have known that the IRB members were doing their jobs. A study this complicated with significant ethical issues takes extra time to review.

- Yes, it's a risky study, but I don't need a sub-investigator. Doctors go on vacation. Doctors get sick. Sometimes doctors just aren't available. This is why the IRB requires the study team to include at least one other physician with the credentials and training to take over if the principal investigator is not available and a study participant needs care.

- We made a mistake that resulted in a protocol deviation. For our corrective action plan, we will re-educate the study team. The IRBs I worked for did not accept this as a corrective action plan. If the error happened after the team received education the first time, the error will happen again unless more action is taken beyond re-education. The IRB wants to see the creation of checklists, the addition of another team member to double check the work, more supervision of support staff such as infusion room personnel, pharmacists, the people checking vital signs, the person responsible for mailing samples, etc.

- You can't leave the research. You signed a consent form. I talked about my experience with this earlier in this book. Everyone on the study team needs knowledge and training on the informed consent process and the rights of research participants.

- I don't care what the consent form says. I always take a biopsy from research subjects. I also discussed this earlier in the book. The principal investigator must ensure that other members of the team know that they must follow the instructions in the protocol. The principal investigator or a designee must carefully review case report forms to look for patterns that might indicate an error like this is occurring.

Consent form readability. In addition to having to educate team members and investigators, I often found myself in situations where I had to educate drug or device companies. I was astounded that I had more knowledge of the federal regulations than the companies who were investing millions of dollars into research needed to get a product approved.

The most common issue I ran into centered on the reading level of informed consent forms. From the first clinical trials I had participated in, I realized the importance of having a consent form that was complete, readable, and organized in a way that allowed participants to find important information if an issue came up. Many of the sponsor template informed consent forms that came from industry sponsors did not meet these criteria. I assumed that they were written by lawyers, or by medical professionals, or both. It appeared the purpose of these consent forms was to protect the sponsor and the investigator from liability instead of to inform the participant of the procedures and risks of the study.

Sometimes, for international studies, it seemed the original consent template had been written in a language like German or Chinese, and then translated into English by someone in Great Britain or India. The syntax would be off in a way that would confuse most participants in the United States. When I was working on helping investigators get translations of English consent forms for their Spanish speaking participants, I had to remind them that Spanish in Mexico, Spanish in Puerto Rico, Spanish in Spain, and many of the other Spanish speaking countries can be quite different. French spoken in France is different from the French spoken in Quebec or in the Louisiana Cajun communities. There is a similar issue with English consent forms intended for use in the United States that were translated in another English-speaking country. United States patients need consent forms translated into United States English.

I learned that my first experience with consent forms from NIH sponsored studies, with the AACTG (Adult AIDS Clinical Trials Group) did not extend to other NIH funded cooperative groups. The AACTG had a standard template for informed consent forms for all studies and used the community representatives to make sure the final consent form was readable. For many of the studies sponsored by NIH funded cancer groups, or cardiology groups, or nursing research, it did not seem like those groups had a process of standardizing consent template formats or ensuring completeness and readability. Instead, it seemed like the investigators had written the consent forms themselves, or had designated someone to write it, with no proofreading by other team members or review by a lay person without a science background.

Sponsors often sent template consent forms that were not in chronological order. The procedures section might start off with the list of tests and number of visits required by the study, and then describe the screening procedures that would have to be done before the participant could start the study. The consent form should describe the screening first. Screening must be completed and passed before the study procedures can begin. Then the consent form needs to say what happens on the day the participant enrolls in the study, followed by the next visit, and the next visit, etc. I was surprised at how many template consent forms did not do this. It made me wonder if the writer was writing in stream of consciousness, listing procedures as they came to mind instead of when they would happen. I would move everything around into chronological order, using track changes and comments to indicate what I moved and why.

Study sponsors did not want me to alter their consent forms. I had to educate my sponsor contacts, through the local study teams, that the federal requirement that a consent process be done in a language the participant could understand did not mean simply to provide English for English speakers and Spanish for Spanish speakers. It meant the consent form needed to use words and sentence structure that would make sense to the participants we were consenting. The flow of the consent form needed to follow the flow of the research procedures. Many of the NIH cooperative groups stated that we could not remove or change the language in a consent form. They would, however, allow me to add explanations and definitions where they were needed. Sometimes they would even let me move some sentences around, as long as I did not change the sentence.

Understanding HIPAA. I had to educate several major industry sponsors about the HIPAA regulations. The most common mistake was the sponsor telling us we had to use their HIPAA language in the consent form, and not the language developed by the legal team and privacy office at our institution. HIPAA applies to the "covered entities." The HIPAA regulations define a covered entity as a health plan, a health care clearinghouse, or a health care provider. In the case of research consent forms, the institution conducting the research is the covered entity. The sponsor can make sure the research clinic is following the HIPAA regulations, but the covered entity has the final word on the HIPAA language that goes into their consent form. The consent form has to explain how the covered entity (the research clinic) will use and disclose the protected health information for research purposes. Our legal team and privacy office must have the final say on what this explanation says.

Understanding emergency use. More than once, I had to educate an industry sponsor on the emergency use of a non-approved, investigational drug. The federal regulations allow for several ways for patients to have access to investigational drugs if they are not able to enroll in a clinical trial for the drug.

- **Expanded access programs** are usually set up when there is a widespread need for a drug that is close to FDA approval, but is not yet available for prescription use. During the early 1990s, a number of AIDS therapies became available to patients who would likely die without the treatment and could not wait another few months for FDA approval. A program like this saved my life.
- **Single patient INDs** allow a drug company, the physician, and the FDA to agree to allow one patient at a site to have access to a potentially lifesaving drug. The drug might not have enough demand to set up an expanded access program like the one described above. For many years, these single patient IND projects would need approval at an IRB meeting before the drug could be used. This meant the single patient IND was only helpful if the patient could wait a few weeks until the full IRB could review the project and approve it at a meeting. Recently, the FDA changed this requirement so that the IRB chair can sign a statement that they concur with the use of the

investigational drug. This allows the patient to receive the drug sooner.

- **Emergency use** is used when the patient needs the drug immediately to prevent death or permanent impairment. A drug to lessen the damage of a chemotherapy overdose needs to be administered immediately. A drug that could treat a life-threatening infection needs to be administered immediately. For situations like these, the federal regulations allow the physician, the manufacturer, and the FDA to facilitate immediate use of the drug to save the patient's life. The IRB must be notified within five days of the use of the drug, and again when the use of the drug is completed. If the patient's life is in immediate danger, the approval of the IRB is not needed before the drug is administered.

Several times I had situations where the physician and the manufacturer had both agreed that a patient was in a life-threatening situation and needed immediate treatment with an unapproved drug. The FDA had agreed to this emergency use. The sponsor would then say they could not ship the drug to our hospital until the IRB approved the use. Because of the likelihood of imminent death of the patient, I would have to place frantic phone calls to the drug manufacturer and read them the federal regulations. I would then have to follow up with emails or faxes describing the rules for emergency use. Meanwhile, my co-workers were busy trying to see if enough Board members were available for an emergency meeting to approve the emergency use if I could not educate the sponsor in time. We could not approve the use in advance of the use unless we could get a quorum in the emergency meeting. In all these cases, the sponsor eventually relented, after consulting with their legal teams. I couldn't help but wonder why an IRB manager at a community hospital had to educate the leaders of an international Fortune 500 pharmaceutical company on the federal regulations for investigational drugs.

<u>Sponsors not providing what the IRB needs.</u> Here is an opportunity for industry education that I encountered frequently. Sponsors often do not provide the sites with new information in a format that the IRB can use. This happens when protocols are amended, when the investigator brochure for an investigational drug is updated, and when there are changes to the risks of the study. The main function of the IRB is to ensure participant safety. The IRB reviewers need to quickly see the changes that affect participant risk. If the IRB cannot easily see the study changes that might affect that, then the IRB cannot do its job. The sponsors are not necessarily violating the regulations, but they are not helping the IRB provide oversight.

If a study is amended, the "summary of changes" document provided the sponsor goes in order through the sections of the study. This is not the summary the IRB needs. Going through the sections of the study, the first items listed might be a change in a member of the global study team, or a change in address for a lab that is running tests for the study. The IRB reviewer first needs to see if anything changes the risks. This could be an expansion of inclusion criteria (we are changing the study to allow persons under the age of 18 to enroll), an increase in the number of x-rays or biopsy procedures, or an increase in the length of time the participant will take the study drug. It could be a newly identified risk of the study drug. In the same way that a good news story starts with the headline, the list of changes for a protocol should start with the changes that directly affect patient safety.

The same is true for changes to the investigator brochure. Sometimes sponsors do not provide a list of changes. When I was the regulatory coordinator for the HIV research clinic, the IRB made me put the two versions side by side and go line by line through many pages to make a note of what had changed. Sometimes a sponsor would provide a list of changes, but the list would include statements like "we have updated the risk list for drug X" without telling what the changes to the risk list are. Again, I would have to go through the risks listed in the old and new versions of the investigator brochure, and identify any new or increased risks, before I could send the investigator brochure update to the IRB.

With consent forms, the sponsor cover letter summarizing the changes usually says "updated risks for drug X." Just like with the investigator brochure, I had to compare the sponsor's consent form templates, the old one and the new one, to see what had changed so that I could report that to the IRB. Sometimes the risk list would be reformatted. This made it even harder to see the risk changes. Comparing the old and new template consent forms could not be done line by line. I would have to look at each risk in the old form separately, and then see if it was still in the newly formatted list. Once I checked off all the risks from the old form, I turned to the new form to see if any risks had been added.

Sponsors not understanding the regulations. I found out that sometimes sponsors and other IRBs are not as concerned as I was about whether my IRB broke a few rules. Once I got a call from the sponsor of a study letting me know that a pediatric oncology patient from my institution had enrolled in a trial in Boston but was back home in Texas now and needed her next dose of the study drug. There was not enough time for me to convene a special meeting before the patient's next dose was due. They asked if we could do an emergency approval of the study. The situation did not qualify for emergency use, though, because the drug was available commercially. The patient could still get the drug outside of the study. The only consequence of having the patient take the drug as standard care instead of under the auspices of the study was that the sponsor could not use the data.

The sponsor suggested that my institution rely on the Boston site's IRB to be the IRB of record. My institution's policy for relying on an outside IRB required approvals at multiple levels of the institution and would take months to complete. The sponsor's IRB director called me and asked me to break our policies and procedures for the sake of the study. Of course, in an audit, the lead site's IRB would be spotless because they hadn't broken any of their own policies. Our IRB, however, would be subject to sanctions in an audit if we broke our policies. My job could also be in jeopardy if I knowingly went against my institution's rules when a patient's life was not in immediate danger. The patient got the drug on schedule but had to leave the research study.

Device companies look for loopholes in the FDA regulations. When I was in Texas, research using the patient's own stem cells was getting a lot of attention, because the Governor, Rick Perry, had mentioned in some campaign speeches that stem cells had sped up his recovery from spinal surgery. At that time, stem cells were only under FDA oversight under certain conditions. If the stem cells came from another donor, they were under FDA oversight. If the patient's own stem cells were used, but they were altered in any way, or if they were sent to an outside lab for processing before the patient received them for treatment, they were under FDA oversight. A Texas company developed a device that would "spin out" the stem cells from a bone marrow sample or a sample of body fat. The device was used in the procedure room where the stem cell harvest and the stem cell injection would take place. The patient never left the room during the harvest and the injection. The stem cells didn't leave the room until after they were injected into the patient for treatment purposes. This kept the whole process out of the jurisdiction of the FDA.

We opened a study that would compare fat cells with bone marrow cells for use in spinal surgery. The study used the in-room device. The study was run poorly. At the time of continuing review, no one at our site could give me an accurate number of how many patients had gotten stem cells harvested and received the stem cells back for treatment. Neither the investigator nor the study coordinator had any records. I called the sponsor. The site was supposed to send before and after x-rays of the patient's spine to the sponsor. I hoped the sponsor could tell me how many x-rays they had received. They could not. They said they did not have all the records on hand. We brought in an outside auditor to check the patient's records for signed consent forms, hoping this would show us how many patients had enrolled. The auditor was able to identify how many records showed a patient had enrolled in the study but could only find two signed consent forms and several blank consent forms in the study records. There was no proof that many of the patients were even aware they were in a research study. I called the FDA. There was nothing the FDA could do because the sponsor had successfully kept the study out of the FDA's jurisdiction. I have seen since then that the FDA has closed this loophole. Our institution shut the study down. Thankfully, we never received any reports of patients who were harmed by the procedure.

When I left the UAB IRB to go to a medical center IRB, I discovered many sponsors were surprised that the local IRB at a medical center was careful in the review of research. Evidently many local medical center IRBs were not as thorough as the IRBs where I worked. Many clinics and hospitals rely on commercial IRBs rather than having their own IRBs. With commercial IRBs, a sponsor can always find one that is a bit looser with the regulations than others.

IRBs and research sites can be their own worst enemies. Sometimes my issues with IRB operations arose from the way the local institution's IRB office operated. The most blatant example was at my first IRB job. I was asked to process study submissions as Not Human Subjects Research when the submissions clearly did not meet the criteria for that level of review. Per the regulations and our own official policies and procedures, the research should have been expedited review or full Board review. I was told that the investigator brought in major grant funding for the institution and held a lot of clout, so we needed to not get on her bad side. She had the power to get IRB staff fired.

At another institution, an IRB member was also on the hospital administrative board and on the state medical Board. He thought the IRB's policies and procedures were too lax even though they were directly from the federal regulations. He felt like the federal regulations were a floor, not a ceiling. Without notifying the IRB administration, he had the hospital Board write their own policies for the IRB. Some of these made compliance impossible. The first thing I did when I found out about this was to create a Policy on Policies for the IRB. The new policy ensured that the IRB had the final say on its own policies and procedures. The policy effectively removed the possibility that one person could impose his own agenda on the IRB.

Sometimes the IRBs where I worked created their own problems, by taking on responsibilities that should have been handled by other departments. In more than one situation, a department at the institution would require department sign off before the IRB reviewed the project. Instead of policing this themselves, the department asked the IRB to check for the department sign off letter before we reviewed the submission. Out of courtesy, the IRB staff agreed to do this. It turned into a bigger burden than we expected, eating up our already overstretched ability to do the work we were charged with. Researchers would turn to the IRB with questions about access to patient records for student investigators, for questions about HIPAA, for questions about hospital policies. The hospitals where I worked had their own departments for record access, their own privacy officer to answer HIPAA questions, and their own policy pages. I would refer the investigators to the appropriate resources. I have learned from colleagues, though, that at other institutions the IRB is the resource for answering these questions and more. Seasoned IRB professionals call this "IRB creep."

Outside regulations impacting IRBs. Other issues ate into IRB resources. At my most recent position, the hospital legal department became concerned about ADA (Americans With Disabilities Act) compliance. This concern arose from a growing trend in our area involving individuals searching web sites to look for non-compliance and then suing the companies responsible for the web sites. The legal bills for these lawsuits were astronomical. Our IRB had posted all our policies and procedures on the hospital web site, along with contact information for the IRB, guidance documents, and frequently asked questions. Without warning, the web site administrators required that we ensure these pages were

ADA compliant, meaning they could be read aloud by a computer audio system so that blind persons could access the information. The first consequence of this was a strain on our time to use online tools to convert all the documents to a format that was ADA compliant. Then we had to wait for someone in hospital administration to certify the compliance. At first, this certification was done at no charge to us. Then the administration outsourced the certification process to an outside company. We had to pay a large fee for each document. We were in the middle of a fiscal year and had no budget for this. Cuts had to be made elsewhere to cover the costs.

In 2009, a new United States President's team decided that medical research would be a priority in his administration. They added millions of dollars to the budgets of federal agencies that sponsor research. These agencies sent out requests for proposals. Medical professionals nationwide were scrambling to come up with research ideas to obtain some of this new grant money. No money was provided to cover the costs of overseeing this new increase in research. Much of the research was minimal risk. I managed the review process for minimal risk research. My staff was cut just as the new research started flooding my inbox. Of course, the NIH had a deadline for the proposals, so all the new submissions were high priority because of the funding that might come to the institution.

One of my professional skills is the ability to make the workflow as efficient as possible. I looked for areas where less important tasks were interfering in my overall productivity. I instituted a "triage" approach. In a crowded emergency department, the staff uses the triage approach to make sure the most serious and urgent cases were handled first. I did the same thing. I had to give highest priority to studies that had the potential to save lives and/or the change medical practice. Lower priority went to those that were primarily designed to advance the investigator's education or career. The ability to generate money for the institution should not have been part of the priority rankings. Sometimes, though, the institution's administration forced me to give these money-making studies highest priority

I realized that one department was putting a major strain on my time because of residents relying on me to teach them how to design a research protocol and fill out the paperwork for the IRB submission and, later on, the IRB continuing review. My first attempt to make better use of my time was to require the department to identify one or two "superusers" among the faculty mentors to train all the faculty mentors, who would, in turn, train the residents they were mentoring. I met with the superusers to train them. The training did not take and did not trickle down. The same questions kept coming in from the residents.

With the help of the rest of the IRB office team, I developed training modules for every step of the research development and IRB submission and review process. I included screen shots for each question on our forms and put in detailed instructions for each. This worked for some investigators, but not for the departments that were causing me the most trouble. I finally had to send out an email broadcast to every faculty mentor in the department, saying the IRB, going forward, would only accept research from their residents if the research was reviewable as Exempt Review or as Not Human Subjects Research. This would eliminate most of the paperwork the residents were having trouble with.

Ideally, I would love to train residents in the regulatory process for research. But the time I spent trying to answer telephone calls and emails, from dozens of residents who did not read the training modules or who could not rely on their faculty mentors, was time taken away from reviewing clinical trials from oncology, cardiology, and other medical treatment areas. The research from these areas had risks that could be life threatening to participants. These projects had to take priority over minimal risk projects done primarily to fulfill a degree requirement.

Impact of COVID-19. All of these frustrations came to a head in early 2020 when our work was disrupted by the COVID 19 pandemic. I am in a high-risk group, so I opted to shelter in place and work from home. At the same time, the hospital was losing revenue due to cancellation of non-emergency surgeries and procedures. The hospital administration needed to make cuts to the budget. The IRB is not a revenue producing department, so we were an easy target. My supervisor asked me to keep a daily log of all my activities so she could prove that I was working and that my work was essential to the hospital. Keeping the log added more burden to my workflow, just as I was getting flurry of submissions and questions about submissions for research on the impact of COVID-19. The hospital had patients who were facing death. I knew I had to triage once again and focus my resources on the projects that had the best likelihood of saving the life of patients battling COVID-19. I created an out of office reply and an email signature to inform anyone contacting me that priority would be given to those projects that could provide medical benefit. I could not get bogged down reviewing and advising on protocols that looked at revenue impacts of COVID-19, or nurses' perceptions of hospital safety guidelines during the pandemic, or whether our hospital sanitation guidelines were adequate. When questions like these came in, I had template language I could quickly copy and paste into a reply email that let the researcher know their project was quality assurance/quality improvement and did not need prior IRB review.

Our medical research team quickly dismissed the few queries we got for doing limited site studies of hydroxychloroquine, which were mainly proposed to get someone a publication credit. They knew that we needed to save our resources for national projects with large numbers of participants, which had the best chance of answering treatment needs quickly. The best prospects for this were remdesivir and convalescent plasma. We were not put on the short list for sites selected for remdesivir. However, the local blood bank was preparing to sign on to a national program for convalescent plasma and wanted to work with us.

At first, there were no protocols in place to streamline the administration of convalescent plasma, which is blood cells from patients who had developed immunity to the virus. The first patients we treated with convalescent plasma each had to be treated under a single patient IND, with an accelerated emergency process to get the product to the patient as quickly as possible. This required several entities to work together quickly. The blood bank, the FDA, the physician, the research department, the research coordinator, the IRB chairman and I each had to work together like a finely tuned machine to get the plasma to the patients before it was too late.

One Saturday morning, I got a text from my supervisor that two of these requests were coming that day. Each of the people I just listed had to work together quickly and efficiently. I contacted to IRB chair to make sure he would stay available so that he could sign off as soon as the paperwork was ready for his approval signature. I contacted the coordinator to make sure she understood exactly what I needed to get the paperwork ready for the IRB chairman. She contacted the FDA, the blood bank, and the physician to make sure they knew their part and were ready to do it. It took all day, but late in the afternoon all the completed documents were on the way to the FDA and the blood bank. At least one life was saved by our efforts. None of this would have been possible if my time had been spent on projects that did not offer the same prospects for immediate benefits.

<u>Need for institutional priorities.</u> Over my career in IRB work, I saw several instances where a major event set off a flurry of protocol submissions. Most of these submissions were done so the investigator could get a publication credit. Many posed little if any prospect of benefitting the public or providing new knowledge. But there was no system in place at the institutional level to prioritize the research and focus resources on the most significant proposals. This happened when a major outbreak of wildfires in south Georgia sent heavy smoke over summer camps in south Alabama. It happened when the local school system bought laptops for all the students in the system to use in class and for homework. It happened after forty-nine people were killed and dozens more shot in a massacre at the Pulse nightclub in Orlando. No one was setting priorities for research after these events. No one was setting up a point person to make sure multiple people weren't trying to do the same research. For the computers for public school students, I contacted the school board president and let him know he had many requests coming. I knew he didn't want his classrooms disrupted by multiple surveys, focus groups, and interviews. He agreed to wait until all the submissions came to his desk and limit the number of projects that would be done in his schools and choose only those that could benefit his schools and students.

When COVID-19 hit, there were three hospital-wide surveys of employee satisfaction. One was from emergency management. One was from human resources and nursing administration. These two were correctly sent to hospital employees without getting IRB approval first. They did not need IRB approval for a team member satisfaction survey. Another was from nursing research. The IRB was asked for guidance on this one, with a plan to send the survey to the IRB for approval prior to administering the survey. All three surveys were asking similar questions to roughly the same group of participants. This happened when everyone's time was stretched to the breaking point.

Within the medical research area, though, the director quickly set up a process for any research proposals to go to his office first. He and his team then selected only the ones that would give the most "bang for the buck." He could also direct the researchers to resources within his department to make the research development go as smoothly as possible, and let the researchers know if someone else was already planning the same or similar research.

6 HOW CAN WE IMPROVE RESEARCH PRACTICE?

- *Instead of doing things the way they have always been done, research could benefit from the example of evidence-based research, and test methods to see which work best.*
- *Too many people are trying to do human subjects research.*
- *Too many sites are conducting research.*
- *Conducting research under the pressure of deadlines can cause errors.*
- *Institutions that require research should compensate researchers for their time.*
- *Research staff should receive better salaries to avoid staff turnover.*
- *Priorities should be set first and used to decide which research will be done.*
- *Everyone involved in research must be capable of critical thinking.*
- *Education is needed, not just for researchers and their staff members, but also for administrators who make decisions that affect the conduct of research.*
- *Degree programs that require a research component must include courses on the conduct and oversight of research.*
- *Board certification in conduct of research should be developed and required for principal investigators of more than minimal risk clinical trials.*
- *Nursing department magnet status should be based on the quality of nursing research conducted, not the quantity.*
- *All research documents, especially informed consent forms, must be at an appropriate reading level and*

written so that the content is clear to the intended audience.

- *The evaluation of risks versus benefits should include looking at who assumes the risk and who benefits financially.*

Evidence based. One trend I have seen in my involvement in research since the early 1990s has been a move toward evidence-based medicine. One of the most harmful statements I hear when discussing change is "But we've always done it this way." Evidence-based medicine challenges this way of thinking. It looks at medical procedures that are common practice but have no data to prove that the procedure actually works, or if other procedures might work better. Evidence-based medicine requires doing research, often comparing a standard practice or a standard medical device with a newer practice or device. The goal of evidence-based research is to make sure we are practicing medicine the best way possible.

I suggest we apply these same principles to how we conduct and manage research. Are we getting the optimal results from current practices? Or are we wasting resources that could be used for projects that have the potential for improving lives? In the last two decades major changes have been made to what had been "business as usual" for research programs. Some have changed from paper based to electronic online methods to handle IRB submissions and correspondence. The system I have used at two hospitals, IRBNet, has improved record keeping and shortened the turnaround time from initial submission to final approval of IRB submissions. Since both the research clinic and the IRB use the same system for research records, we no longer have to spend hours making sure the site records and the IRB records for a study are the same when the study is audited.

Because the system is online, requests for more information or for corrections, and the study teams' responses, can be handled in less than a day, instead of waiting for paper requests and responses to go through campus mail. The IRB reviewers post their comments and requests online before the meeting. I can make sure these are addressed before the IRB convenes to vote on the submission. In almost all cases, I have been able to send out approval documents on the day the IRB met and voted. This is the electronic system I am familiar with. I know there are other programs available for electronic IRB submissions and records, that have helped other research sites.

At the same time, research sponsors have been moving toward more online record keeping and reporting with the research sites. Research sites and medical clinics are converting to electronic records. All these changes have cut costs and improved efficiency. In some cases, the change to electric records have simplified the process for retaining records. At one IRB where I worked, the multiple filing cabinets holding paper research records became so heavy the building engineer made the IRB move many of the records to another site, because the floor for the IRB offices was in danger of collapsing into the offices below. That IRB is now busy converting those files for electronic storage.

Another change is the use of central IRBs to review a study at several sites. Commercial IRBs were created starting over fifty years ago to serve as the IRB of record for research sites who did not have the resources to create their own IRB. Over the years, these commercial IRBs became the IRB of record for multiple sites doing the same study, so that the study sponsors did not have to send the same study to multiple IRBs. Each IRB has its own forms and its own policies and procedures. Switching to a central IRB made the IRB review process more efficient and less costly for sponsors. In the last two decades, the FDA and OHRP have issued guidance assuring sites that using a Central IRB does not violate federal regulations. Recently, the NIH began requiring multi-site studies funded by the NIH to use one IRB as the "single IRB" for the study at all sites. <u>These examples prove that research programs are capable of major changes and can benefit from them.</u>

Below are some "sacred cows" that I believe need to be looked at and challenged to see if changing them can improve research practice.

<u>Too many people are trying to do human subjects research.</u> Currently, it seems that everyone who gets an advanced degree or everyone who wants to advance their career must do research. Many of these have no desire to be researchers. They only want to do be the best that they can be in their chosen field. Hospitals, medical practices, and academic institutions should take a hard look at whether the requirements for research are meeting the goals of the requirements. Does being a researcher mean you are a better doctor, nurse, social worker, pharmacist, or costume designer? Are there better ways to measure professional achievement?

The ever-growing requirement for research means the committees that oversee research are overburdened with reviewing many projects that have little chance to benefit the general public. Hospitals need nurses who are excellent nurses. Hospitals need doctors who are excellent doctors. There needs to be enough research to support this excellence. Select the few who want to be researchers and are willing to do the education and work to become excellent at research. Let the others benefit from their skilled and focused work.

I recommend removing the "publish or perish" mantra, and instead find other ways to recognize and retain excellent employees. For students who need a research project to become a nurse or doctor or pharmacist, encourage projects that will improve their skills at their chosen profession, rather than improving their skills at research. A future cardiologist might do "library" research on how a certain medical practice, like using stents in heart disease treatment, was developed and refined. This might be more useful, to students who will eventually use that practice as professionals, than conducting a satisfaction survey of cardiologists who use stents, for the sole reason of demonstrating the student's statistical skills.

<u>Research is conducted at too many sites</u>. Conducting research at too many sites can mean there is less oversight from the sponsor, from the FDA, and from the IRB or IRBs that are reviewing and approving the research. Resources for oversight can easily be stretched too thin. Sponsors sometimes use many sites to speed up enrollment. Involving community representatives in the design of the research could accomplish this goal while reducing the expense of opening many research sites.

Research conducted at independent "research centers" may suffer from lack of oversight by a hospital board or a local IRB. I have friends who have worked at some of these free-standing research centers. They report that good clinical practice often suffers. The centers are likely paid by the number of patients enrolled and/or the number of patients who complete the study. Without oversight, it is easy for the researchers at these centers to bypass inclusion criteria and enroll patients who should not be enrolled, or to gloss over adverse events or unexpected problems in order to keep patients on a study who should be removed.

Sponsors often choose this kind of clinic to conduct their research because they know they can get data to support the treatment they are trying to get approved without having to worry about following too many regulations. This focus on making money instead of patient safety has resulted in harm to study participants.

The FDA publishes a regular summary of warning letters sent to researchers. A high percentage of these warning letters are sent to independent researchers or research centers. I recommend that the federal research regulatory agencies take a hard look at where and how research is conducted and consider limiting medical research to sites that meet tougher standards.

I recommend that sponsors and the FDA look at their current policies for certifying research sites and selecting sites for research. Limiting research to sites with proven records of good clinical practice and protection of human subjects will benefit the patients and the sponsors. It will also help ensure public confidence in medical research.

Do deadlines result in poorly designed research? As I write this book, I see headlines (https://www.washingtonpost.com/health/2020/06/04) about a published article being retracted from the Lancet, a major medical journal. In the retraction (https://www.thelancet.com/journals/lancet/article/PIIS01 40-6736(20)31324-6/fulltext), the editors state that there were concerns about the veracity of data and the data analysis in a study conducted by Surgisphere Corporation. The Surgisphere founder, Sapan Desai, was a co-author of the article.

The initial publication of the study showed major risks in using hydroxychloroquine to treat COVID-19. The published article was based on an analysis of existing data on the use of hydroxychloroquine in the treatment of COVID-19. This was not a randomized clinical trial. It was a review and analysis of existing data. As such, my best guess is that the IRB that approved the study used expedited process rather than full Board review, since the risks to patients were minimal from the data collection and analysis.

Lancet asked to do an independent audit of the data, but the study team would not release all the information. They stated that patient agreements and confidentiality concerns prevented them from doing this. Without this data, the Lancet could not conduct the independent audit to verify the results found by the Surgisphere research team. News reports about the retraction blame the study team for rushing to get the publication done. The Lancet is criticized for not adequately reviewing the article before publishing it. I have not seen any criticisms of the IRB yet. I imagine the IRB likely did not spend a lot of time reviewing all the details of the project before approving it, due to the minimal risk and the pressing need for information on treatments for a growing pandemic.

Unfortunately, the use of hydroxychloroquine became a political football. One side advocated its use and even bought up large supplies of the drug to use to treat a condition with no conclusive proof that the drug would work, and little information on the risks involved in using the drug for this condition. The other side wanted more caution and more proof of safety and efficacy before the drug was used on a large scale to treat COVID-19. There were known risks of hydroxychloroquine from the research done to get it approved to treat other medical conditions such as Lupus. These risks have the potential to be more serious in people with COVID-19, based on information on how COVID-19 affected those who became seriously ill.

The retraction of the Lancet article only showed that there were concerns about the data analysis and that the concerns could not be addressed. It did not disprove the findings. It only said the findings were not well supported. We still do not have conclusive evidence, based on this study, on whether hydroxychloroquine is safe to use in COVID-19 patients. One side of the political spectrum is taking the retraction as an excuse to yell "fake news" and state that this means the use of the drug is risk free. The other side is pointing to articles from randomized controlled trials that show little benefit of the drug in the treatment of COVID-19. They state that even without knowing for sure if there are additional risks for COVID-19, there are risks. Why take those risks in a drug that has no benefit?

The political element that is driving this debate means time and resources are being taken away from finding treatments that will have benefit, with fewer risks. The rush to get something published, by the study team and the journal, worked against the goal of finding the best way to handle the pandemic. It also led to even more distrust of the scientific community in a time when we need scientists to lead the way.

The above is an example of why requiring research for degree requirements and career advancement may lead to bad research. The rush to be the first to publish something about the hot topic of the day can do the same. Students, medical professionals, and tenure-track faculty have deadlines to meet so they can move forward. Forcing research into deadlines created by arbitrary dates that have nothing to do with the goals of the research increases the chance of errors. These errors can cause significant problems for all of us. Even in a minimal risk chart review study, questions about the reliability of the results can have significant adverse impacts to the advancement of science and patient care.

How can we improve research? I saw one possible answer at my last IRB job. Several departments at that hospital have a highly trained designated mentor for the residents who are doing research. Instead of setting a deadline that the research must be completed before the residency ends, the mentors have set up a process by which residents roll off the research projects when their residency ends and new residents are rolled into the projects when their residency starts. For more complex studies, the mentors make sure a qualified statistician works on the data analysis. Results are not published until the team is sure that the analysis is complete and can stand up to peer review.

Doctors are required to do research but are not compensated for their research time. At UAB, physicians in the research clinics received part of their salary from the grant money they brought in to conduct research. This grant money also paid for the nurses, data managers, regulatory coordinators and others who served on the study team. This was not the case at the two hospitals where I worked. The hospitals wanted to be known as research hospitals, so they required departments to do research. Even though the industry sponsored research studies brought money into the institutions, the physicians who conducted the research did not get compensated for the time spent on research patients. Physician pay is based on how many non-research patients they see. If research patients take time away from paying patients, the physician's salary goes down.

The physician investigator signs a document saying that they will be responsible for the conduct of the study. The person responsible for the study should have time to supervise the work of the rest of the study team. But the requirement to conduct research without compensation to the research investigators means there is less time to make sure each member of the study team is doing their job correctly. The investigator has to trust that each one is trained and ready to do their job. But without time to do the training themselves, the physician must assume that the study sponsor or a research operations department will conduct that training. This leaves too much room for errors to occur, especially in complicated studies. If a hospital wants to be a research hospital, the hospital administration needs to back that up with enough funding and infrastructure to ensure that the research can be done correctly.

Research errors and failures reflect on the whole hospital, not just the research program. A news article about the FDA shutting down research, or the hospital being sued for a research error that resulted in harm, can have a significant impact on the willingness of the local population to come to that hospital for medical care.

Inadequate pay for research staff. At both hospitals where I worked, I continually had to explain to human resources and hospital administrators what an Institutional Review Board is and what my job entailed. I assume that the clinical research coordinators, research data managers, and research managers ran into the same issues. If human resources and hospital administration don't know what we do, and the importance of what we do, how can they adequately fund our programs? Because of the low pay, I saw a constant stream of people who worked in research staying at the job just long enough to become productive, and then getting hired away by a drug company, a medical device company, or a contract research organization for significantly higher pay.

<u>Setting priorities for research and doing research that fits into these priorities.</u> Earlier in this book, I described my experience as a community advocate for the national Adult AIDS Clinical Trials Group (AACTG). This group was responsible for major improvements in AIDS treatment that were developed and approved with record setting speed. They were able to do this because they set research priorities. They included the AIDS community in the priority setting process. Then they made sure their resources went to clinical trials that would best support these research priorities.

When Bill Clinton was in his first term as President, the First Lady, Hillary Rodham Clinton, was charged with developing a plan to overhaul the United States healthcare system, to provide better and more affordable medical care to everyone in the USA. When Congress began hearings to debate the plan, the congressman from my district came to Birmingham to meet with stakeholders and hear what they needed. He met with pharmaceutical companies, with insurance companies, and with hospital administrators. He did not meet with any patients. I was, at that time, on disability with AIDS, and having trouble navigating the health care system even with insurance. The voices of people like me were never heard, at least not in my district. The plan developed by First Lady Clinton ultimately failed to become law. Had patients been consulted, lawmakers may have looked more favorably on the proposed changes. At the very least, the impact of the patients, who are also voters, could have been used to put pressure on the politicians.

When setting priorities for research, patients must be included. This is the only way to ensure that the research will help develop medical practices that result in the best possible care. If patients help set research priorities, you increase the odds that the studies will enroll quickly, speeding up the timeline for completing the research. Even drug and device companies sometimes seek input from patient community advocates when developing research. I was part of a community group that met several times with drug companies that were developing research for new treatments for HIV, Hepatitis B, and Hepatitis C. One company wanted to exclude people of African descent from a study on an HCV (Hepatitis C Virus) treatment. We convinced them that the study would be more ethical and scientifically valid if these patients were included.

Priorities could be set at the national level, by the National Institutes of Health, by the Centers for Disease Control, and by professional organizations for specific types of medical care. With professional organizations, the American Medical Association could take the lead. Organizations for specific areas of medicine, such as cancer, endocrinology, cardiology, radiology, nursing, informatics, and others could follow suit and set research priorities within their areas. At the local level, hospitals could set their own priorities for research. The hospitals where I worked set annual goals such as reducing hospital-borne infections, safely reducing inpatient times, reducing re-hospitalizations, improving patient satisfaction, and reducing hospital deaths. These annual hospital goals could easily become part of the hospital's research priorities. When any entity sets priorities, it is a good idea to rank them, and to include slots for "late breaking" and "other."

A hospital might set a priority of emphasizing research that can directly benefit patient care. Another hospital priority might be research that reduces costs or does not require expanding hospital resources. The physicians might want to do Phase I research, to give the researcher and the hospital the prestige of doing cutting edge research. But Phase I research is not designed to treat patients. It is designed to make sure the treatment is safe, and to determine the highest dose that can be administered without too much harm to the study participants. By this design, some patients will not get enough treatment to do any good, and others will get too much treatment, resulting in harm.

Phase I research also requires hiring more staff, both in the clinic and in the IRB, because these studies are complicated, often require inpatient care and frequent monitoring for adverse events and are frequently amended because of the newness of the treatment. Frequent amendments mean more work for IRB staff and IRB members. If the hospital research stakeholders, including the patients, set a priority of doing cutting edge research to increase prestige, then the hospital administration needs to fund the infrastructure to ensure that Phase I research is conducted safely. However, if the hospital's research priority is to conduct research that can directly benefit patient care, they may decide to let other institutions conduct the Phase I research.

Within a medical area, like oncology, input from patients on research priorities might include finding treatments with less severe side effects, or seeing if treatment can be enhanced and the impact of side effects can be reduced by alternative treatments, like music therapy, art therapy, or healing touch treatments. Research priorities like these could result in studies that include professionals from other departments, like nurses, chaplains, rehabilitation professionals, and therapists. Instead of each of these areas doing their own research projects, they could all work together on one project.

If a national organization like the National Cancer Institute or the American Society of Clinical Oncology had set similar research priorities, the study could be conducted at multiple sites nationwide, increasing the likelihood that the study results could improve medical practice. A resident or student who needed a research credit could be part of a local research team for this national study, instead of having to create their own research project.

With recent NIH requirements that federally funded studies must use one IRB for all sites, the work burden and costs for most local IRBs would be reduced. At hospitals where I have worked, if an investigator decided they wanted to do Phase I research, there were no research priorities in place to help the hospital administration and research make a decision on whether to allow the research to move forward. These decisions were made on a case by case basis, rather than being part of a master plan. I believe that all research stakeholders, including hospital staff and patients, benefit more if there are priorities to follow.

If a hospital decides to set research priorities, they may apply differently to sponsored or multi-site research than to local investigator-initiated research. For sponsored and multi-site studies, the research department, if faced with two proposals aimed at the same condition and/or the same patients, might give an edge to the proposal that most closely matches the hospital's priorities. Since these studies originate outside the local institution, the hospital's priorities would go into effect once the sponsor starts looking for sites to conduct the study.

For local investigator-initiated research, the priorities could be more proactive. In mid-year, the hospital's research agenda committee, or similar group charged with setting priorities, could finalize the research priorities for the next year. Once these are set, they could be published in the intra-agency web sites and newsletters, or in mass emails to individuals and teams likely to propose research in the coming year. A request for proposals might be sent, with a deadline for proposal requests. When the requests come in, the committee could give the go-ahead for those projects that most closely match the institutions priorities for the coming year.

If multiple proposals are submitted for the same condition and/or the same patients, the teams could be encouraged to work together on one study, rather than having both studies continue. The examples I gave in the previous chapter shows the redundancy in research that could be prevented by having a research oversight committee that sets priorities and chooses research projects accordingly. Reducing redundancy helps budget resources within the institution and increases the odds that the selected studies can accomplish their goals by not having to compete with others for the same participants. The research oversight committee would need to work with the institution's administration to ensure that the budgets and staffing projection are consistent with the needs of the prioritized research. They will need to be reminded that cutting edge research and higher risk research require larger budgets to cover more dedicated team member time and more work volume for the IRB staff and IRB members.

At the national and global level, the NIH and NIH funded consortia, along with professional organizations, could set national priorities for research needs, sending requests for proposals that match these priorities. As proposals come in, the team that reviews the proposals could encourage that individual sites work together in multi-site studies, rather than each site doing its own thing. This would not only save resources, it would also create more meaningful statistics with a better chance, if applicable, to create improvements in patient care and institutional policies and procedures. Team leaders could be encouraged to choose research sites that are best suited for each project when choosing sites for the multi-site study.

Remember that industry sponsors, like drug and device manufacturers, set their priorities based on potential sales. Their priorities are market driven and based on serving the company stockholders. Federally funded and investigator-initiated research priorities should be based on the needs of the patients being served. Market driven research responds to trends. Company A is making money from this treatment, so we need a treatment that will capture a piece of this market. Federally funded, non-profit grant funded, and investigator-initiated studies should create the trends rather than responding to the trends. Their resources need to go for medical needs that are unmet, rather than competing with an effective and safe treatment that is already available.

Setting priorities for research, and choosing the best research to meet these priorities, must come from the research community or the institution's administration. During the years when I was managing IRBs, I saw several instances where the research community wanted the IRB to set the priorities and limit redundant research. Investigators asked me to persuade the IRB not to approve a competing study. IRBs do not have the authority to do this. They can only review and approve each study based on its study design, scientific merit, and risk to benefit ratio.

<u>Critical thinking.</u> In my earlier career teaching costume design at the college level, I worked at three universities, each with different student populations. One class I taught was Introduction to Theatrical Design. In the semester, students learned the elements of design and the connotations each have. Then they learned how to analyze a play to determine themes that the designs would need to support. Colors like black and deep red, combined with sharp angles and rough textures, can help support themes of murder or anger in a play. Soft colors and textures can help support themes of love and kindness.

Once the students had learned the design elements and the basics of play analysis, I had them apply these. I selected Macbeth as the play since most students had some exposure to Macbeth. Students analyzed the play and identified themes. We discussed possible themes in class. Then I asked individual students about design elements that support these themes. "What colors could be used in the design of Macbeth to support the themes we identified?"

At the private university, with high entrance requirements, I immediately got responses. "I would use black in the designs to reflect death." "I would use red in the designs to support the emphasis on murder and stabbings." "I would use sharp angles to suggest the evil and violence in the play." There is not just one correct answer to the question. All of these were correct answers, because the students had used critical thinking to apply the principles to the play to answer the question.

I got similar responses at the university where most students were working full time and took classes at night. In their jobs, they had already learned how to practice critical thinking.

At the state university, the students looked at me blankly when I asked the question about what colors to use. Finally, one student raised her hand meekly. "Is black right?" I responded: "Why would you choose black? What elements in the play will black represent?" The student took her hand down. "Never mind." The students had all done well on the exams for design elements and play analysis but could not take the next step of using critical thinking to apply what they had learned.

When I discuss the need for more education in research, I am talking about more than just memorizing the definitions and regulations and policies and procedures. If you know how to use Google to look up a definition or a regulation, you don't need to memorize it. Short courses, if done right, can at least give an overview and teach students how to find information. Teaching a short online course is easy. The team member passes the course, and the IRB can check off the requirement for training for that person, meeting the FDA requirement for "trained" researchers and research personnel. Even the certification exams for clinical research coordinators and IRB professionals seem to focus on memorizing facts, history, and regulations. Is this enough?

When I talk about needing more education, I am talking about the need to teach stakeholders in research conduct how to think critically about how to apply the published regulations, policies and procedures to everyday decision making. A short webinar or online course cannot do that. You need at least a semester to go through the basic principles and then use hypothetical cases or real-world examples to develop the skills to use critical thinking to solve complex research problems. Institutions must either require this kind of training for all researchers and research teams or provide funding to hire professionals to make up for the lack of education in the research teams. This needs to be done on the research side, and not the IRB side. Asking the IRB office to teach critical thinking is like asking an IRS auditor or and IRS policy maker to help taxpayers fill out their tax return forms.

Education needed for the people who decide the budget. The cost to hire and train a new person to replace the one who left is much higher than increasing the salary of the person who is already on the team. One solution I offered was to educate all hospital employees, especially Human Resources and hospital administration, on the importance of research and the importance of having highly skilled research and IRB team members. Both hospitals where I worked had mandatory training for new employees to cover major components of hospital operations. Neither would agree to give time to the research program. Not only did this meant that the ones holding the purse strings did not know what research teams did, it also meant that there were many employees at the hospital who did not know they needed IRB review and approval before they did research. My supervisors often asked me for documentation on my workload, so they could justify my salary. Continually having to prove that my job was important did not build a sense of my job security or my engagement in the institution. Research can be improved if hospitals include the research department as a necessary and valuable component of hospital operations, on equal standing with medical departments, marketing, human resources, housekeeping, conference services, and others.

Several times while I worked at a community medical center, I heard administrators say the institution needed to decide whether it was a research center or not. If we were a research center, then there needed to be funding to support the research infrastructure so that we could do the research correctly. I contend that this applies to education about research. Every year when I worked in a hospital, I had to take training on patient care and patient safety. My job did not involve any direct interaction with patients. Neither did the jobs in payroll, human resource, maintenance, budget and finance, and many others. We all had to take the patient care and safety courses because we worked in a hospital. The same needs to apply if the institution decides to become a research center. If so, then everyone in the institution, including administrators, needs education and training on how research is conducted and what regulations govern institutions that conduct research.

Training for researchers and research staff must be added to degree programs. Medical students, nursing students, pharmacy students, and others who are required to do research almost always have to take courses in statistics to complete their degree requirements. Why are there no requirements for courses in research regulations and research oversight (IRB) requirements? Many of these institutions rely on the IRB staff to do this training. IRBs are not funded to do the amount of training required to teach a potential researcher all they need to know. At my last IRB job, our hospital allowed students and faculty from a nearby university to do research in our facilities. I continually reminded my supervisors and the department heads at the university that I was not part of the university faculty, and not being paid to teach their students and faculty.

Every degree program that requires research projects should require courses in managing research, and understanding and applying research regulations, the same way they require courses in statistics. Few, if any, academic institutions have courses like this in their curricula. They must be created and added. Lack of this training leaves the would-be researchers stranded and frantic when they need to get their research approved and then conduct the research. The regulations are too complicated to teach in an hour-long seminar, an online course, or in the IRB staff's spare time. Even a full semester of training can barely scratch the surface. The education process must include case studies and analysis to help teach the process of using critical thinking to solve problems. The textbooks that are developed for these courses could be a foundation for self-driven continuing education for these students.

Residency programs should require courses like these as prerequisites for being assigned to a residency. Currently, the faculty mentors overseeing the residents are supposed to provide this education. In my experience working in a research clinic and in IRBs, most of the mentors do not have the knowledge to provide this education. Either they don't do research, or haven't done research in a long time, or, if they do research, they have a research team including a team member who handles all the regulatory requirements.

When I was a regulatory coordinator, I was not allowed to take more than a few minutes to help a resident with an IRB question. This is not enough. It should not fall on the clinic staff to provide training that the residents should have gotten during their formal education. At my last job in a IRB office, I tried to get the hospital's medical education department to help support a full time employee to handle this training, since the residents were not getting it from their schools or from their mentors. I never got a response. I finally developed some online basic training tools as a stop-gap measure to help the residents.

At that job, I also got asked to help train new team members for the various departments doing research. While I was there, I was able to work with the research department to set up experienced clinical trial coordinators in positions designed to do this training. We required all team members to pass online CITI courses in research ethics, privacy, and good clinical practice. Many of the job descriptions required board certification from professional societies like SoCRA (Society of Clinical Research Associates.) The IRB staff is required to obtain Certified IRB Professional status through a program under PRIM&R (Public Responsibility in Medicine and Research) as soon as they meet the minimum time working at the IRB. These certifications require work experience and a passing score on an extensive exam. They could serve as a model for principal investigators, faculty mentors, and others charged with training students, fellows and residents in conducting research.

Even with these certification requirements in place, though, I still found that many of the team members who did IRB submissions struggled with our web based IRB system, and did not know how to answer many of the questions that were required for IRB review. I planned to create an online course for these team members and for the entire research community, including students, residents, fellows and their mentors. The course would contain modules for each step of the IRB submission process. Each module would have questions that must be correctly answered before the user could move on to the next module. I hoped the institution would support requiring a passing grade on the course before anyone could send in an IRB submission. With the help of the other IRB team members, I created the training modules. They were based on existing training documents we had in place and on training documents provided by the company running our online IRB submission system. I put all the information in chronological order, added definitions of terms, and included screen shots of the online submission program to provide visual aid into the education. Each module had questions for review at the end.

I beta-tested the modules and questions by using them when questions came in on how to send something to the IRB. For most researchers and team members, the training modules successfully answered their questions. They were able to complete their submissions without one on one instruction from me. This freed me to spend more time doing my job of preparing submissions for IRB review and approval. If I had not retired, my next step would have been to turn these modules into the online course that researchers and research team members would have to pass.

<u>Should Board Certification be required to conduct human subjects research that is more than minimal risk?</u> This question was posed at a breakout session at a PRIM&R Advancing Ethical Research (AER) conference a few years back. Many areas of medicine encourage or require Board certification. At many research sites, other members of the study teams, such as clinical research coordinators, must have Board certification. Most institutions will not hire an IRB administrator unless the applicant is a Certified IRB Professional or is eligible to take the exam to get that certification. Why not researchers?

Above I have made a case for across the board training in research regulations and local research oversight requirements. Research investigators, especially the Principal Investigators (PIs), must be skilled in many other areas. A PI is responsible for all facets of the conduct of a research project. At the UAB HIV research clinic, the PI for most of the studies gave excellent oversight. At our weekly research meetings, he knew the duties of each member of the research team and was able to effectively oversee our work and advise us on processes.

Not all researchers are that hands-on. Once I started working in IRB offices, I realized that most researchers let the Clinical Research Coordinators run the studies. If a document needs signing, they don't review it, they just sign it. Then they are surprised when an audit or inspection reveals misconduct or extensive protocol deviations. Some of this lack of oversight may be remedied by providing pay for the time a medical professional conducts research. But that won't be enough if the investigators do not know what they are supposed to do.

I envision a certification process which would ensure knowledge of all relevant regulations and ethical considerations, and how to apply these. The certification for a principal investigator could require the applicant to first serve as a sub-investigator on a minimum number of clinical trials. The certification for sub-investigators could require the applicant to complete and pass a full semester course in research regulations and managing research.

The certification exam for PIs and sub-investigators should include testing to make sure the applicants know how to follow study procedures of a complicated research protocol, especially if the procedures differ from standard practice. It should test for the ability to discern when an unanticipated event (protocol deviation or adverse event) occurs. Applicants must prove they know the difference between a major event and a minor event. They should show that they know the requirements for reporting these events.

There could be an additional education and training

component for this. Physicians must do a residency for several years to specialize in areas like cardiology, radiation oncology, or infectious diseases. For those physicians who choose to conduct more than minimal risk research, a residency program in research could be required as part of or in addition to the Board certification.

Research institutions could set this standard. I could not apply for a job as an IRB administrator without my Certified IRB Professional (CIP) Board certification in place or close to completion. Would-be researchers could be held to this standard.

Research sites compete for selection to conduct high profile research. If a site tells the sponsor "all our investigators are Board certified to conduct clinical trials" the odds would increase for that site to be selected as a study site. Clinical trials consortia, like the Adult AIDS Clinical Trials Group, the Children's Oncology Group, the National Heart, Lung, and Blood Institute, and others, could set the same requirements. The time to train investigators on a study could be reduced. The number of deviations in the conduct of the study could be reduced. This could streamline the time to complete the study. If the goal of the study is FDA approval, the improvements in study conduct could enhance that process.

<u>Basing nursing Magnet Status on the quality of research rather than the quantity of research.</u>
"Magnet status" is an award given by the American Nurses' Credentialing Center (ANCC), an affiliate of the American Nurses Association, to hospitals that satisfy a set of criteria designed to measure the strength and quality of their nursing. At the sites where I worked, the nurses seeking magnet status for the hospital spent a lot of resources on

increasing the number of research studies done by nursing staff. I hoped the team that conducted the inspections for magnet status would consult with the IRB about the training level of the nurses and the quality of the research projects that were submitted, but they did not.

If Magnet is measuring the strength and quality of nursing, and using research as part of that measure, the inspectors need to look closely at the research projects that are done. I think the strength and quality of nursing is best served by nursing research projects that have a positive impact on patient care or reveal more efficient, cost-reducing ways to improve nursing care without sacrificing quality. Many critics have stated that working for Magnet status uses valuable hospital resources but adds little to quality of patient care. Better selection of research and quality improvement projects could change that perception. The team that awards Magnet status should include this as part of their site evaluation, including interviewing the IRB members who review nursing research submissions.

<u>Require a minimal readability level for all informed consent and assent forms.</u> Early in this book, I discussed my struggle understanding the language in research consent forms for studies I enrolled in. I am highly educated and test high in scales of reading comprehension. I still had difficulty understanding language written by medical professionals and legal advisors. In the early 2000s, some NIH cooperative groups tried to set a standard for the reading level and length of informed consent forms. Risks of treatments and procedures the participants would have, even if they were not in the research study, were moved to appendices at the end of the consent form, leaving the informed consent form risk language to focus on the risks unique to participation in the study. I saw a few attempts to conform to these new guidelines. However, most study teams preferred to stick with their standard processes for writing consent form.

When the first draft of proposed changes to the Common Rule were issued in the early 2010s, it included a requirement that consent forms meet a set standard for readability. After several years of comments and discussions, these new standards were removed. The final regulations retained the previous statement that research must be conducted in a language that the participant could understand. For institutions that were concerned about readability, the IRB staff was usually charged with rewriting the informed consent forms.

An IRB member I worked with for several years insisted that all research informed consent forms be edited to a score of eighth grade level or lower on the Flesch-Kinkaid readability tool. This tool evaluates readability by looking at word length, sentence length, paragraph length, and active versus passive verb tense. This is a good start, but it does not address all the issues in readability. This is another area where critical thinking should be applied. It is not enough to reach a score on a scale that only measures sentence length, word length, paragraph length and verb voice. These things may be in place in a consent form that is still hard to read and understand.

I think informed consent forms should be written in language that reflects the way people talk. Almost nobody says "prior to" in ordinary conversation. They say "before." They don't say "you will have some of your blood drawn." They say, "Go to the lab and the lab tech will draw some of your blood." They don't say "in the event that you should happen to be injured due to your participation in this research." They say "if you are injured because of a study procedure." When I review and edit informed consent forms, I make sure that my neighbor, my niece, and my friend who works at the grocery story could understand the form if they were enrolling in the study. The sponsors should be doing this before the template consent forms go to the sites. If not, the study teams should do this. If the IRB staff members are the only ones ensuring readability, the institution should consider this when budgeting the IRB staff.

Federal regulations state that minors are not old enough to provide consent. Their parents or legal guardians must consent for the minors to participate in research. The regulations also require an "assent" process for much research that included minors. An assent process ensures that the minor participants are aware of why they are being asked to take part in the research and what will happen in the research study. The regulations only require an assent process. Most institutions, though, require the minor's signature on an assent form, to document that the assent process took place. IRBs where I have worked made sure the reading level of the assent form was appropriate for the age of the minors involved.

The evaluation of risks versus benefits could be expanded to include looking at who assumes the risk and who benefits financially. Recently, there was discussion in the media about a novel plan to speed up the development of a vaccine for COVID-19. Normally in a phase three vaccine study, hundreds of patients are given either the experimental vaccine or a placebo. All are counseled on the best ways to avoid infection. Participants who enroll are in good health but may be at risk of infection due to factors in their daily life. Over time, the group that received the experimental vaccine is compared with the group that received placebo. The research team looks to see if there is a statistical difference in how many participants in each group became ill with the disease the vaccine is intended to prevent. They measure the number of people in the placebo group who became infected despite using standard precautions to prevent infection. Then they look at the numbers from the group that received the experimental vaccine. They see how many got infected despite receiving the experimental vaccine and taking standard precautions. If the numbers are the same as the placebo group, the team can assume the vaccine does not work. If there are no infections in the vaccine group, this proves the vaccine works. If there are some infections in the vaccine group, but fewer than in the placebo group, this likely means the vaccine is partially effective. All the participants must be followed over a length of time to get these results.

The novel plan to speed up the approval process involves intentionally infecting all study participants with the COVID-19 virus. Participation in the vaccine study would be limited to those with low risk of becoming seriously ill from the infection. Not waiting for participants to be exposed by everyday life would produce comparison data much faster. Intentionally infecting the participants, instead of waiting for the virus to take its natural course through the population, would dramatically reduce the time to determine if the vaccine works.

Many question the ethics of intentionally exposing participants to a potentially lethal or debilitating disease. If there is a placebo group, everyone in the group would likely get infected. If the vaccine did not work, or only worked for some participants, then all participants would be at high risk of infection with a dangerous disease.

Some proponents argue that the risks are necessary for the good of society. Having to wait for many months for standard research to prove the efficacy of a vaccine could mean thousands of lives lost in the absence of an effective vaccine. This raises the ethical question of whether the lives of a few should be sacrificed for the good of the rest of us. I wonder if Russia was able to license a vaccine so much quicker than other countries by using this "intentional exposure" method.

Proponents of the intentional infection plan also said that the participants would receive generous compensation for the risks they were taking. My first thought was: "How generous?" The drug company that manufactures an effective vaccine against a disease like COVID-19 stands to make billions of dollars in profits. These profits would be passed on to company executives and stockholders. None of these people would be risking their health or their lives. How much payment should the participants receive for assuming these risks? How can this plan be made ethical?

I propose that studies like these be done by nonprofit and government funded entities, rather than by private industry. If, however, private industry proceeds with a study that uses intentional exposure, then caps should be placed on the cost to the public who will take the vaccine. If the company wants to speed up the process for the good of society, the drug must be affordable to everyone in that society. If the cost of the vaccine is significantly higher than the manufacturing costs, this makes it seem that the real motivation is profit, and not societal benefit.

Allowing drug companies to make billions of dollars from intentionally exposing study participants to harmful disease is not consistent with the medical principle "First, do no harm." This principle is part of the Hippocratic Oath, taken by all medical students. Intentionally doing harm, when motivated by profit, rather than the possible benefit to society, compounds the violation of this oath.

My doctor has asked me if I am interested in enrolling in a COVID-19 vaccine study at his clinic. I will look closely at the informed consent form to see who is sponsoring the study and what kinds of risks I will have if I enroll.

In this chapter I have offered suggestions for ways the practice of research can be improved. There may be others. I close this chapter the way I began it, with this sentence: One of the most harmful statements I hear when discussing change is "But we've always done it this way."

7 SHOULD YOU ENROLL IN RESEARCH?

- *Is your current care working?*
- *Do you want to help others?*
- *Who is the sponsor?*
- *Are there any "red flags?"*
- *If you do enroll, what is next?*

Because I have worked in medical research and have served as a research community advocate, I sometimes get asked by groups and individuals for my opinion on whether I recommend enrolling in a research study. Here some of the points I use to make decisions like this for myself.

Is my current care working? There is an old saying, "If it ain't broke, don't fix it." I look at whether the medicines I am taking are doing their job. Is my blood pressure lowered? Is my cholesterol within recommended levels? Is my HIV undetectable? If not, this may be a reason to look for a better treatment that might be available in a clinical research study. Then I look at side effects. Even if the medicines are working, are they harming my body in other ways or reducing my quality of life? There may be clinical research studies for drugs that are designed to reduce these side effects. Sometimes for me, finances are what is "broke." I recently retired. The copayments on my AIDS medicine, under the Medicare Advantage plan I enrolled in, are quite high. In addition to looking at financial assistance, I am also looking for clinical research studies that might offer HIV medications at no cost to me.

Do I want to help others? There may be research studies that offer little or no benefit to me but might help improve future treatments for me and for others. If the study does not pose much risk to me, I might enroll in the study to "pay it forward." The medicines I currently take were developed through clinical research. That research depended on volunteers to get the results needed to bring the medications to market. I welcome the chance to do the same for others.

Sometimes I am asked to take part in a survey study or complete a questionnaire for a research study that will help a medical resident advance their career or a student complete the requirements for a degree. If I have the time to help, I usually do. We need more doctors, nurses, and other professionals to keep entering the work force as others retire. If I can help the new ones get started, I am glad to do that.

Who is the sponsor? Should I worry about who is sponsoring the study? While the impact on the results may be different for industry sponsored studies and for government funded studies, this should not affect the potential risks and benefits to the study participants. I talk about interpreting research results in the next chapter.

Are there any "red flags?" I have a few criteria that I use to evaluate research studies. I look at how much the study participants will get paid. If the payments are unusually high in relation to my time and inconvenience for participating, it might be because the risks of the study are unusually high.

I look at the risks lists in the informed consent form for the study. Some of these risks are risks I would have anyway, even if I did not take part in the study. Some may be more severe but have a low chance of occurring. I look for risks and side effects that are likely to happen and are unique to the study.

Once I was recruited for a research study that used a treatment called IL-2 to see if it could boost the immune response to HIV. A common risk of IL-2 is feeling like you have the flu for a few days after each treatment. The treatments were every two weeks. My current health was stable. I looked at results from other immune response studies in HIV and did not see many signs that they worked. Because of the likely risk of flu symptoms every two weeks, I did not enroll in the study. I discuss risk lists in more detail in the next chapter, Interpreting Research Results.

I was recently asked to consider enrolling in a COVID-19 vaccine study. One of the listed risks is that I might still get COVID-19 if I take the vaccine being studied. In addition, for this experimental vaccine, my symptoms, if I do later catch the virus, might be much worse than if I did not get the vaccine. I decided not to participate in this study.

Another red flag I look for is future access to the treatment if it helps me while I am in the study. Some research studies have this built into the study design. For some, if there is a placebo group, the participants who initially receive placebo will have the option of crossing over into the treatment group at a specified time. For many Phase III studies, the sponsor promises what is called a "rollover study" for participants who have seen benefit in the Phase III study. This gives them continued access to the drug through a research study until the FDA approves the study for marketing.

For Phase I and II studies, I ask if participation in the early phase studies will keep me from taking part in the Phase III studies. This happened to a friend of mine who enrolled in a Phase I study for a drug designed to treat HIV in a different way from approved drugs. My friend saw significant health improvement while on the study. The study only lasted a few weeks. When the sponsor started the Phase II and III studies, they excluded any patients who had already been exposed to the drug. It took several years for the manufacturer to open expanded access programs that allowed my friend to resume the drug that had helped him.

In general, I advise people to study the consent form and ask questions. The regulations require that you have as much time as you need to make a decision about enrolling in a research study. You have the right to ask a medical professional, a trusted friend, or a family member to help you decide. If you are consenting on behalf of your child, you should also look at the assent form that your child will sign and ask the study staff to make sure they explain difficult concepts to your child. Encourage your child to ask questions.

I've decided to enroll in the study. What do I do now? Here are some of the steps I have taken when I have enrolled in a clinical research study:

- I studied the informed consent form. I looked at it again before each study visit. I tried to make sure that nothing happened to me in the study that I had not agreed to.
- I kept a copy of the informed consent form. For some studies, I took it with me to study visits, and referred to it when meeting with the study team.
- The informed consent form includes information on who to call if I have problems or questions about the study, and who to call if I have questions about my rights as a research participant. I put this information where I could find it quickly. With today's technology, I would put the information into my smart phone.
- I kept track of any new symptoms, and reported them to the study team immediately, especially if they were serious.

- If the study did not provide tools to make sure I was taking the medicine as prescribed, I developed my own tools, like a calendar or a daily checklist.

8 PRODUCT LABELS AND RESEARCH RESULTS

- *Sponsors can manipulate the data to skew the meaning of the results.*
- *Can limited data be useful?*
- *How are the risks determined? What do they mean?*
- *Recognize the positive spin on research results.*
- *Who is the sponsor of the study?*
- *Where was the study conducted?*
- *Look at the study design.*
- *Did participants know what treatment they were getting?*
- *Beware of news releases for "promising new treatments."*
- *Where were the results published?*
- *What if a respected journal publishes study results and later retracts the article?*

<u>Manipulating the data</u>. Mark Twain said: "There are three kinds of lies: lies, damned lies, and statistics." In the case of research results, there is a fourth category, misinformation or "not exactly a lie." The reason statistics get a bad rap is that they are so easily misinterpreted and can be manipulated to look like they are proving a point. Interpreting research results is important and requires education on how to look critically at the information.

For FDA regulated products, the label and the marketing must reflect the results of the FDA regulated research. Even for products that do not fall under FDA oversight, the label and advertising cannot make false or unproven claims.

Most of us see research results on television ads for products.

Listen carefully to how the words are used. You may hear something like "clinically proven to reduce the appearance of wrinkles." This is likely a cosmetic. Cosmetics are not regulated by the FDA. There is no government agency to confirm any research results. "Clinically proven" can mean anything from a full-blown clinical trial where some participants got the cosmetic and others did not, to a manufacturer using the cosmetic on a few people and saying: "your skin looks younger."

There may be photographs to back up the claim. If you look closely, the before and after pictures likely don't have the same lighting on the person's face.

The clue that this is a cosmetic and not a drug is in the phrase "reduces the appearance." Only a drug that has gotten FDA approval can make a claim of medical benefit. If the ad said the product reduced wrinkles, that would imply a medical benefit. The FDA has the authority to stop unproven claims of medical benefit.

For cosmetics, you often see celebrities saying: "It works for me. It can work for you." Yes, maybe it can. But no one can promise that you will get the same benefit as Eva Longoria, Cindy Crawford, Blythe Danner, or any other celebrity. To prove the likelihood of benefit, there must be a controlled clinical trial, comparing a statistically significant number of people who get the product with a statistically significant number of people who don't.

The same is true for nutritional supplements and aromatherapy products. These are not normally classified as drugs, so the FDA can only intervene if false claims of medical benefit have been made. If an energy drink or an essential oil company makes a claim that their product has been clinically proven or says: "studies have shown," you should find out about the studies. Ask how many people were in the studies and whether there was a comparison group. In Chapter 2 of this book, I describe a nutrition supplement study I took part in. This was likely not under FDA oversight, even though the goal of the study was to see if the new product would help patients with AIDS wasting syndrome. As long as the supplement was not marketed as a cure or a treatment, it would fall into the category of nutrition supplement and not an FDA-regulated drug.

I currently drink a product called Boost Glucose Control Balanced Nutritional Drink. I have it every day with breakfast. The label for the product is carefully worded. It does not claim that the Boost Glucose Control controls blood sugar levels. It says it is "designed for people with diabetes." It says: "To help manage hunger." It says: it is "specifically designed for people with diabetes to help manage blood sugar levels as part of a balanced diet." Finally, it tells me "it's clinically shown to help manage blood sugar levels vs. a standard nutritional drink in people with Type 2 diabetes."

What does all this tell me? First, it tells me this is not an FDA regulated drug. Even though the product name has "control" in it, the label does not promise cure or control. It tells me this may help if used along with a balanced diet. Most important for me, it tells me there was some kind of comparison made with another popular nutrition drink. It does not tell me which nutrition drink.

The label does not claim to be better for diabetics than any other nutrition supplement. It only states that diabetes management was better with the Boost product when compared with one other nutrition drink. The most important information on the label, for me, is that one serving contains twenty-two grams of protein and one gram of sugar. It has no dietary fiber, but it does contain vitamins and minerals. Part of my plan to manage diabetes is to reduce hunger so I am not tempted to snack too much. The drink does that for me, even if it is a placebo effect. It also satisfies my daily craving for chocolate, with only one gram of sugar.

The same kind of language can be used for FDA regulated drugs, even if the deception is not intentional. A doctor in the United States southwest gave hydroxychloroquine to all his COVID-19 patients. They all recovered. He claims this is proof the drug works. It is an indicator that the drug might work, but it is not proof. Unless he gave a placebo or another treatment to some of his patients, made sure there were enough patients in each group for statistical significance, and compared the results from the two groups, he has no proof that the recovery was due to the drug. Unless the results are much better from the group that got the drug, then you can't prove the drug made a difference. The patients likely would have recovered from COVID-19 without the drug. Later studies did use this comparison model and found no improvement. The study results seem to conflict. The misinterpretation of the results causes this apparent conflict. Yes, the doctor's patients did get better. But this is not proof of benefit yet.

Similar confusion is seen in the analysis of side effects for hydroxychloroquine. Many pointed to the FDA-approved use of the drugs in other conditions like lupus, saying that the side effects for these people were acceptable. There are two fallacies in this interpretation. The first is revealed if you note that clinical trials had been done showing that there is medical benefit to patients with lupus who take hydroxychloroquine. There may be serious risks of the drug, but they are outweighed by the benefit to the reduction of the effects of lupus. The second fallacy is in comparing side effects for one disease with side effects for another disease. COVID-19 has a different impact on the body than lupus. Certain body systems and organs become more vulnerable to the side effects of hydroxychloroquine, making the side effects much more severe. A drug with an acceptable risk to benefit ratio for one disease may not be acceptable for another disease. This is why the drug information that comes with your prescriptions tells you what conditions (indications) the drug is approved for.

The debate on using hydroxychloroquine to treat COVID-19 became political. This caused even greater confusion over what the results mean. It also raised suspicion on both sides of the political spectrum over how drugs are tested and approved. Mark Twain was talking about politicians when he made his statement about "lies, damned lies, and statistics."

Can limited data be useful? In some situations, it may be useful to know that a drug might work, even if it is not proven. In the early 1990s, I was diagnosed with a serious lymph node infection called Castleman's Disease. There are not enough cases of the disease in the world to conduct a statistically valid study on any potential treatments. My doctor looked in medical journals for case reports. A case report is a published article about a new approach to an unusual condition or disease that was tried in one patient or a very few patients. The case report includes the patient's outcomes. My doctor explained to me that he wanted to try some treatments that were not proven to work but had worked in one or two other patients. The first treatment he tried did not work and had serious side effects that could have permanently damaged my kidneys. With the second treatment my symptoms did improve. These case reports provided valuable information that helped my doctor treat my disease. They did not prove that the treatment worked, but they offered options to try.

Developing risk lists for drugs, devices, and procedures. Informed consent forms for research studies are required to include a section on the risks of the study. For minimal risk studies, the risks section might simply say that there are no anticipated risks to participants, or that the only risk is possible breach of confidentiality. For studies using drugs, devices, and/or diagnostic procedures like x-rays or CT scans, the risks must be listed. These risk lists are developed based on the results of earlier research. Study team members must interpret the data on side effects and adverse events and determine if the risk lists need to be revised. Risk lists are constantly updated based on interpretation of study results.

For FDA approved drugs, the product label or package insert also includes known risks of the treatment, based on all the research results and on risks discovered after the drug was approved for use. You might see some of these risks flash by quickly in the television ads for the approved drug. Understanding the risk lists requires knowing how they are developed.

Before the research in humans begins, some possible risks can be inferred from looking at the results of research in animals, or results found in the lab, or risks of similar drugs. If the study is Phase I, and has not been tested in humans, the first informed consent might only include these risks or may list fewer risks. Remember that one of the purposes of Phase I research is to find out more about risks and determine the maximum amount of drug that can be administered before the side effects become unacceptable.

As the treatment or intervention is used in human patients, in the current study and future studies, the study team and sponsor collect all information on any side effects or unexpected adverse events. These may be added to the risk lists. Sometime the adverse event may be caused by the drug or device or it may be caused by other factors like diet, exercise, environment, other medications the study participant is taking, or by the disease being treated. For example, in HIV research, no one with HIV can be given just one drug. One drug therapy, or monotherapy, in HIV can lead to the virus quickly mutating to become immune to the drug. All AIDS and HIV patients must be on more than one drug. If a study participant develops headaches or nausea, it may be hard to tell which drug is causing this. The risk gets added to the risk list for all the drugs the participant is taking. HIV and HIV treatments are associated with conditions like high blood pressure, high cholesterol, metabolic changes like changes in body shape, and certain infections that are not normally seen outside of the HIV/AIDS population. Notice that I wrote "associated with." It is hard to prove if the HIV or the HIV treatments caused these conditions, but they are common or more common in patients living with HIV and taking HIV treatment.

If you add a new study drug to a participant's list of medications and they develop high blood pressure or metabolic changes, is this caused by the new study drug, or by the progression of the HIV disease? Research investigators are asked to evaluate whether they think the condition is related, probably related, possibly related, or not related. Unless they can completely rule out (not related) the role the study drug may have played, the condition usually gets added to the risk list. Some informed consent forms may provide the frequency of the side effect or adverse event has occurred. Sometime risks may be rare. Sometimes the side effect occurs in almost all patients.

When I look at a risk list, I compare it to my own medical history. If a drug may cause diarrhea, I know that I have a history of having this side effect with many drugs. I weigh the possibility of more diarrhea with the possible benefit of the study drug. Since I know from experience how to handle diarrhea, I usually do not let this keep me from enrolling in a drug study. If a drug can cause a rare severe allergic reaction, I let the investigator know which drugs have given me a severe allergic reaction in the past. The investigator or a research pharmacist may know if the study drug is similar to a drug I am allergic to. When I was approached for a study using IL-2, I was told that almost everyone has flu-like symptoms for a few days after receiving the drug. I did not enroll in the study. Almost all informed consent forms say there may be other risks that are not known yet. Participants are urged to tell the study team if they have any new symptoms or side effects. Their information could help refine the risk list for the study treatment.

Drug companies put a positive spin on data. Drug companies want to sell their drugs. This is part of our economic system of capitalism. This does not mean the drugs are harmful. It means that the study results will be presented in the best possible light to increase sales. An advertisement for a new cancer drug may say or imply that it will extend your life. To better understand the study results, ask how long the average patient's life will be extended. It might be two months. It might be several years. Then look at the side effects of the drug. Most ads list these. If the drug is likely to only increase your life by two months but you will be miserable with side effects for those two months, it may not be worth it unless you only want to live long enough to see your daughter get married in five weeks. If the drug increases the life of most patients by several years, with minimal side effects, it might be worth your time to discuss the drug with your doctor, your pharmacist, and your insurance company.

The television ads for drugs show happy people climbing mountains, taking dance classes, or directing an outdoor theatre company. Before you assume you will be that active if you take the drug, talk to your doctor about your current medical condition and how much benefit you can expect from the drug. Since some doctors receive payment for administering drugs, you may want to get a second opinion from another doctor or a pharmacist.

Who is the sponsor of the study? Since drug companies present study results in the best possible light, find out who sponsored the study. If the study was sponsored by the manufacturer, keep that in mind while you are looking at the study results. Read between the lines. What information is missing? If the study was sponsored by the NIH, or by a grant from a government agency or non-profit, there is less likelihood that the results will be sugar coated to make the drug or treatment look better.

Where was the study conducted? You may find this information by searching www.clinicaltrials.gov. It may be part of the news release on the drug's approval. A simple google search may lead you to published articles about the research, which may include the sites where the study was conducted. I put more faith in research done at respected research institutions than I do for research conducted at small local research-for-profit clinics. If I cannot find out where the study was conducted, I assume the study sites are not respected research institutions.

Look at the study design. The published study results should tell you if the study included a comparison group that did not receive the study drug. This is the most reliable way to show that a drug makes a difference. I also try to find out how many people participated in the study. Higher numbers mean more reliable results. If the drug is being compared with another drug instead of a placebo, then higher numbers of participants may mean that they needed a lot more data to prove that the study drug was as good as or better than the comparison drug.

Did participants know what treatment they were getting? "Placebo effect" means that you feel better if you think you are getting treatment, even the product you take does not include any active ingredients. The best way to prove the drug makes a difference is to make sure the participants and the study team do not know who is getting study drug and who is getting placebo. This is called a "double-blind" study.

Beware of news releases of "promising new treatments." As someone living with AIDS, I notice the news reports that say scientists have found a promising new treatment for HIV. I've seen a new "promising treatment" at least once a year since 1990. If I don't see the news release firsthand, my relatives and friends will call, text, or email me to tell me about it and ask me if I am going to take the new treatment. Very few, if any, of these ever get past the initial phases of drug development. They are not yet treatments. They are not promises. They are ideas with limited potential. The news releases go out to boost interest in the manufacturer and possibly boost the company's stock value. They are aimed at investors, not the public. Unfortunately, they create false hope in patients who have the disease, resulting in later disappointment.

<u>Where were the results published?</u> I am most interested in study results published in respected medical journals. These journals require peer review, which means scholars in the same field look at the results and agree that the article should be published. These reviewers look at study design, statistical analysis methods, data integrity, and whether the results can be reproduced. If the results are only posted on social media, or in journals with little or no scholarly credentials, I do not take them as seriously. Before I dismiss the social media reports, I try to find reliable sources that confirm or disprove the claims.

<u>What if a respected journal publishes study results and later retracts the article?</u> It is easy to assume that this means the drug didn't work after all, or the side effects did not occur as reported, or the data was misinterpreted. I try to find out why the article was retracted. If it was retracted because the review process was rushed, or the data analysis was incomplete, this does not mean the information in the article was incorrect. It means the process was not complete enough to support the claims in the article. If politics are involved, as we saw in the debate over a study on side effects of hydroxychloroquine when used to treat COVID-19, the news of the retraction of the article can be used to create even more misinformation. I try to consult several sources to try and find the truth.

9 EPILOGUE: COVID 19

I first heard about a new virus outbreak on the other side of the world in late 2019. Over the next few weeks, I watched and read the news to see the slow spread of the virus around the world and inside the United States. I watched local leaders in Central Florida, panicked at losing tourism dollars, going on television news to proclaim that the Orlando area was still open for business. When Walt Disney World, six miles from my house, closed its gates, I knew it was time for all of us to take the virus seriously. The suggestions I had been making for improving the research process became even more important.

Setting priorities. I knew from experience that an event of this magnitude would generate many ideas for research projects. I also knew that the resources of the IRB office and of the research department at my hospital would be stretched as far as possible. We all began putting priorities into place

My first step was sending a general announcement to researchers that I would be giving highest priority to reviewing research with life saving potential. This priority would apply to new research and to continuing review and amendments for current research projects. The priority applied to research related to COVID-19 and to research on the other areas of medicine at our institution. I added a similar statement to my Outlook email, as an automatic reply and as part of my default email signature.

The research department set up similar priorities for which COVID-19 projects they would support with research staff and for how current research would be conducted while participants were required to shelter in place and avoid close contact with others.

I knew that the IRB would be approached with small scale investigator-initiated studies on possible treatments for the virus. I felt that with our limited resources, we needed to focus on participation in large scale, national projects with the potential to quickly identify treatments that would work. I found out soon that research administration had set similar priorities. We began working with a local blood bank and the NIH to set up a means to deliver convalescent plasma (blood product containing antibodies to COVID-19, donated by survivors) to our patients with the most urgent need. The first few of these were done by using the emergency use process, since we had not yet been added to the national protocol for convalescent plasma use.

The physicians who would be administering the convalescent plasma had limited training in opening a clinical research project. Since we could not wait for the training to get done, highly trained and experienced members of the research administration team stepped up to take over the correspondence with the FDA, the NIH, the blood bank and the IRB. I talked with my supervisor about ways we could streamline the IRB submission and approval process, since every minute was important. The IRB chairman agreed with our plan. We were able to get emergency use plasma to three patients within hours of the request from the physicians. I was glad I had communicated to other researchers that anything not related to saving lives would not get first priority. I spent hours doing my part in the approval process for this emergency plasma use and advising others on the team what they needed to do. Everything else coming into my office had to wait.

Research administration knew we could not sustain the extra work required to get emergency use approval for convalescent plasma to all our patients who needed it. They focused their efforts on quickly getting our site approved to participate in the national protocol. I agreed with leadership that we should defer oversight to the central IRB for the protocol. This saved us the several days or even weeks it might have taken to get local IRB approval. Approval of the protocol at our site would speed up the process for getting plasma to individuals whose life might depend on it, since the approvals would already be in place. The all-day process of getting emergency use approval was no longer needed.

When I had the chance, I looked at other submissions for new research. Two of these, from nursing research, fell under the category of "quality improvement" and did not need IRB review. I urged the researcher to start her projects quickly since they could have an immediate impact on measuring our hospital's response to COVID-19 patients, including the impact on front line workers and the effectiveness of our standard infection control procedures.

Our site tried to get added to the national protocol to test Remdesivir as a possible treatment for COVID-19. We were not chosen as a research site. But within a few days, the NIH took an unusual step and issued a blanket emergency use approval for using the drug for COVID-19 treatment. My hospital was able to administer the drug to patients who needed it. Since this was not research, involvement or approval by the IRB was not needed. This helped us get another treatment to patients quickly.

At the national level, priorities for responding to COVID-19 were affected by politics. Political leaders promoted a drug already approved for other diseases. There was no proof that this drug would be effective in treatment of COVID-19. There were known risks of the drug when used for other diseases. Research studies showed the side effects and risks were even greater when treating COVID-19. While there were reports that some patients saw improvement after treatment with the drug, later studies that compared the drug with placebo did not show any benefit. If politicians had not insisted on using the drug, and making it a partisan issue versus science, valuable time and resources would not have been wasted.

Another facet of my hospital's response to COVID-19 involved how to conduct current research while under social distancing restrictions. Leadership responded quickly with guidelines for deciding which research to put on hold, which research could be conducted remotely with "virtual visits" and how to ensure the safety of participants in studies that involved treatment and/or needed face to face contact for safety testing.

Need for education. Our hospital was fortunate to have trained research leaders to step in to help get approvals for the investigational drugs our patients needed. In an ideal world, the physicians would have also gotten that training. This might have helped speed up the process a bit.

The COVID-19 pandemic also showed the need for hospital leaders and administrators to know more about the research process and the need for trained personnel on the IRB team. At the same time work increased due to the added pressures of the pandemic, research team members and IRB team members were having to account for every minute of each workday as part of a process to prove our work was necessary. When hospitals run short of funds, research is often the first area considered for elimination to cut costs.

Even while I documented that my work was saving lives, I worried that I might be the next person laid off.

<u>Moving on.</u> In late May, I was offered a generous early retirement package. Retirement would start on June 6, 2020. The hospital system was losing millions due to reduced patient contact. They needed to cut costs. Hospital administrators decided the most painless way to do this was to offer early retirement to team members in good standing who were old enough to qualify for Medicare and either at full retirement age or close to it. For various reasons, including fear of losing my job later and fear of having to stop social distancing and return to work in a hospital before the pandemic was over, I decided to retire. I had been making notes for this book for many years. Now I would have the time to write it.

Recently, I was asked to screen to take part in a research study of a vaccine for COVID-19. If I qualify and decide to sign the informed consent form, I will once again be a research participant. If I participate, it will be with the knowledge gained from being a participant in other research, from being a community advocate for research, from working in a research clinic, and from managing the Board that oversees research.

ABOUT THE AUTHOR

Harry C. S. Wingfield has a unique view of Human Subjects Research (Research on People). He has been a research participant, a research participant advocate and activist for AIDS research at the national level, worked in a research clinic, and was a senior staff member for three Institutional Review Boards, the committees that approve and oversee Human Subjects Research. He holds an ABJ (BA in Journalism) from the University of Georgia, where he graduated magna cum laude, Phi Beta Kappa. He also holds an MFA in theatrical design from the University of Texas at Austin. He is the author of Closets: A Memoir with Music, which tells his story of coming out as gay in the 1970s, struggling with addiction and alcoholism, becoming a gay rights activist, singing at Gay Pride rallies all over the country, and surviving AIDS. He has also written two plays: Open Discussion, a musical set in a Texas LGBTQ Alcoholics Anonymous group, and Gratia Plena, a ten-minute play about AIDS survivor guilt. He is currently retired and lives in Davenport, Florida near Walt Disney World.